EAT
TO
HEAL

A Practical Guide to Nourishing Your Body
and
Treating Disease Through Food

Eat to Heal – A Practical Guide to Nourishing Your Body and Treating Disease Through Food

1st Edition

Story concept and text © 2025 by Kevin B. DiBacco

Cover design © 2025 Amidei Arte.

Editing, print preparation, formatting, back cover summary, and final cover design © 2025 Amidei Arte and © 2025 Staback Author Services.

Books may be ordered through popular, online retailers, Page Turner Books, Inc.'s online store, or by contacting the publisher at:

Page Turner Books, Inc.
222 N. Lafayette St., Suite 11
Shelby, NC 28150

Visit our website at www.ptbooksinc.com or contact us via email at contact@ptbooksinc.com. Page Turner Books, Inc.'s name and logo are copyright of Page Turner Books, Inc.

iBook ISBN: 978-1-967289-24-0
Kindle ISBN: 978-1-967289-25-7
Hardcover ISBN: 978-1-967289-22-6
Paperback ISBN: 978-1-967289-23-3

Printed in the United States of America. First Printing: September 2025

ATTENTION CORPORATIONS AND ORGANIZATIONS:

Most Page Turner Books, Inc. books are available at quantity discounts with bulk purchase for educational, business, or sales promotional use. For information, please call or write:

Special Markets Department, Page Turner Books, Inc.
222 N. Lafayette St., Suite 11, Shelby, NC 28150
Telephone: (702) 606-1775

EAT
TO
HEAL

A Practical Guide to Nourishing Your Body
and
Treating Disease Through Food

Kevin B. DiBacco

Shelby, North Carolina, USA

I want to thank my Soul Mate, Rachel, for all her support and encouragement.

I truly thank Leanne and the crew at Page Turner Books, Inc. for believing in this book and my future projects!

TABLE OF CONTENTS

INTRODUCTION
THE SCIENCE BEHIND FOOD AS MEDICINE

Now, I know what you're thinking. "Food as medicine? Sounds a bit woo-woo.' But stick with me here because the science backing this up is mind-blowing.

Let's start with inflammation. You've heard this term thrown around a lot, but what does it really mean? Well, inflammation is your body's natural response to injury or infection. It's like your internal emergency response team. Short-term inflammation is a good thing. It helps your body heal. But when inflammation becomes chronic, that's when problems start.

Here's where food comes in. Certain foods can either promote or reduce inflammation in your body. For example, a study published in the *Journal of the American College of Cardiology* found that people who ate a diet high in red and processed meats, refined grains, and sugary beverages had higher levels of inflammatory markers in their blood. On the flip side, those who ate plenty of fruits, vegetables, whole grains, and fatty fish had lower levels of these markers.

But it's not just about inflammation. The food you eat can influence your genes. Yeah, you heard that right. There's this fascinating field called nutrigenomics that looks at how nutrients can turn certain genes on or off. For instance, research has shown that compounds in broccoli and other cruciferous vegetables can activate genes that protect against cancer.

And let's not forget about our gut microbiome—the trillions of bacteria living in our digestive system. These little guys play a considerable role in our health, influencing everything from our immune system to our mood. The food we eat directly impacts the composition of our gut microbiome. A study published in the journal Nature showed that switching from a plant-based diet to an animal-based diet changed the microbial composition in the gut in just 24 hours.

iii

What to Expect from This Book

So, what can you expect from this book? Well, buckle up, because we're going on a journey through the fascinating world of food as medicine. But don't worry—this will not be some dry, academic textbook. Think of it more like having a chat with your gym buddy who happens to be a nutrition nerd (guilty as charged.).

We're going to cover a lot of ground, from the basics of how food impacts your body at a cellular level to specific dietary strategies for common health issues. We'll explore different eating approaches, debunk some popular myths, and give you practical tips for incorporating healing foods into your daily life.

Here's a sneak peek
at what's coming up

The Science Behind Food as Medicine

We'll dive deeper into how what you eat affects your body, right down to your DNA. Don't worry, I promise to keep the science talk fun and easy to understand. No PhD required.

Nutrients 101

Get ready to become best friends with proteins, carbs, fats, vitamins, and minerals. We'll break down what each one does for your body and where to find them in delicious, wholesome foods.

Gut Health—Your Body's MVP

Trust me, your gut is way more important than you might think. We'll talk about how to keep it happy and why that is essential for your health.

Food for Specific Health Conditions

Whether you're dealing with heart issues, brain fog, chronic pain, or a wonky immune system, we've got you covered. We'll explore how tweaking your diet can help manage these conditions and more.

Popular Diets Demystified

Keto, plant-based, intermittent fasting—we'll cut through the hype and look at the pros and cons of each approach.

PRACTICAL TIPS FOR EVERYDAY EATING

Let's face it, knowing what to eat is one thing, but doing it is another. We'll talk meal prep, eating out, dealing with cravings, and more.

Throughout the book, I'll be sharing stories from my experience and from clients I've worked with over the years. You'll see how real people have used food to overcome health challenges, boost their athletic performance, and just feel better.

REAL-LIFE SUCCESS STORIES

Let me tell you about Sarah, one of my clients. Sarah came to me feeling exhausted all the time, struggling with her weight, and battling constant bloating. She'd tried every diet under the sun, but nothing seemed to stick. We started by focusing on whole, nutrient-dense foods and identifying some potential food sensitivities. Within a month, Sarah's energy levels were through the roof, her bloating had subsided, and she'd lost 10 pounds (4.54 kg) without feeling deprived. But the best part? She told me she finally felt control over her health.

Or take Mike, a fellow powerlifter who was dealing with chronic joint pain. We tweaked his diet to include more anti-inflammatory foods like fatty fish, berries, and leafy greens, while cutting back on processed foods and sugar. Not only did his pain improve, but he ended up setting a new personal record in his next meeting.

These are just a couple of examples of the transformative power of food. Throughout this book, you'll hear many more stories like these, showing you the real-world impact of the principles we'll be discussing.

MY APPROACH TO FOOD AND HEALTH

Now, I want to be clear about something: this book isn't about pushing anyone's 'perfect" diet or telling you that you need to completely overhaul your life overnight. As a trainer, I've seen firsthand how unsustainable those approaches can be. Instead, we're going to focus on making small, manageable changes that add up to big results over time.

And here's something else I want you to keep in mind. While food can be incredibly powerful for healing and prevention, it's not a magic bullet. If you're dealing with serious health issues, it's crucial to work with healthcare professionals. Think of the strategies in this book as complementary to, not a replacement for, conventional medical care.

Alright, so why should you listen to me? Well, beyond my background in athletics and training, I've spent years studying nutrition, attending conferences, and working with experts in the field. But more importantly, I've walked the walk. I've used these principles to transform my health and the health of countless clients. I've seen people go from struggling with chronic pain to running marathons, from battling constant fatigue to having energy to spare.

But you know what? You don't have to take my word for it. As we go through this book, I encourage you to try things out for yourself. Experiment with different foods and approaches, pay attention to how your body feels, and find what works best for you. Because at the end of the day, you're the expert on your body.

THE EVER-EVOLVING WORLD OF NUTRITION SCIENCE

I'm also going to encourage you to keep an open mind. Some of what we'll discuss might challenge what you think you know about nutrition. That's okay. The field of nutritional science is constantly evolving, and part of the excitement is learning new things and adapting our approach as we go.

For example, remember when eggs were considered bad for your heart? Well, more recent research has shown that for most people, eggs can be part of a heart-healthy diet. A study published in the *American Journal of Clinical Nutrition* found that eating up to 12 eggs per week had no negative impact on cardiovascular risk factors in people with pre-diabetes and type 2 diabetes.

Or how about the idea that all fat is bad? We now know that certain types of fat, like those found in avocados, nuts, and olive oil, are beneficial for our health. The famous *PREDIMED* study indicated that a Mediterranean diet supplemented with extra-virgin olive oil or nuts significantly reduced the risk of major cardiovascular events.

These are just a couple of examples of how our understanding of nutrition is constantly being refined. Throughout this book, we'll be looking at lots of current research and scientific studies. But don't worry—I promise to break it down in a way that's easy to understand and, dare I say, even fun. No falling asleep with your face in the book, I promise.

WHAT THIS BOOK IS (AND ISN'T)

Now, let's talk about what this book isn't. It's not a diet book in the traditional sense. You won't find any strict meal plans or calorie counting here. It's not about losing weight (although that might be a side effect for some people). And it's not about deprivation or giving up all the foods you love.

Instead, this book is about empowerment. It's about giving you the knowledge and tools to make informed choices about what you put into your body. It's about understanding how food can be your ally in achieving optimal health and performance. And yes, it's about enjoying delicious, satisfying meals that just happen to be good for you too.

As we go through this journey together, I want you to think of food not just as fuel but as information for your body. Every bite you take is sending messages to your cells, influencing how they function. Pretty cool, right? Once you start viewing food through this lens, it can completely transform your relationship with eating.

WHO THIS BOOK IS FOR

I know what some of you might be thinking. "But I'm not an athlete. I'm just a regular person trying to feel better and maybe lose a few pounds." Well, guess what? The principles we'll discuss apply to everyone, whether you're a competitive powerlifter or a busy parent just trying to keep up with your kids. Good nutrition is the foundation of health for all of us.

Throughout the book, I'll be sharing plenty of practical tips and strategies that you can start implementing right away. We'll talk about how to stock your kitchen for success, how to make healthy choices when eating out, and even how to satisfy your sweet tooth without derailing your health goals.

And because I know life gets busy, I'll also share some of my favorite quick and easy recipes that pack a nutritional punch. Trust me, you don't need to be a gourmet chef to make healing foods taste great.

The Journey, Not the Destination

One thing I want to emphasize is that this journey is all about progress, not perfection. In my years as a trainer, I've seen too many people get discouraged because they couldn't stick to a super-strict diet 100% of the time. That's not what we're about here. We're aiming for sustainable changes that you can maintain long-term, not a quick fix that leaves you feeling deprived and miserable.

Remember, every healthy choice you make is a step in the right direction. Today it's adding an extra serving of vegetables to your dinner. Tomorrow it's swapping out your usual snack for a more nutrient-dense option. These small changes add up over time, and before you know it, you're feeling better than you ever thought possible.

I remember working with a client, let's call him John, who was initially overwhelmed by the idea of changing his diet. We started small by just adding a piece of fruit to his breakfast. Then we gradually added more vegetables to his lunch and dinner. Before long, John was naturally gravitating towards healthier choices, simply because he felt so much better when he ate them. That's the kind of sustainable change we're aiming for.

The Joy of Eating

As we wrap up this introduction, I want to leave you with one final thought. Food is one of life's great pleasures, and nothing in this book is meant to take away from that. In fact, I hope that by the time you finish reading, you'll have an even greater appreciation for the incredible variety of delicious, health-promoting foods out there.

I want you to get excited about trying new foods and recipes. I want you to experience the satisfaction of nourishing your body with wholesome, delicious meals. And most of all, I want you to feel empowered to take control of your health through the choices you make every day.

So, are you ready to dive in? Great. Let's get started on this exciting journey to better health through the power of food. Trust me, your body (and taste buds) will thank you.

Remember, you've got this. And I'll be right here with you every step of the way. Now, let's turn the page and start exploring the wonderful world of food as medicine. Get ready to transform your health, one delicious bite at a time.

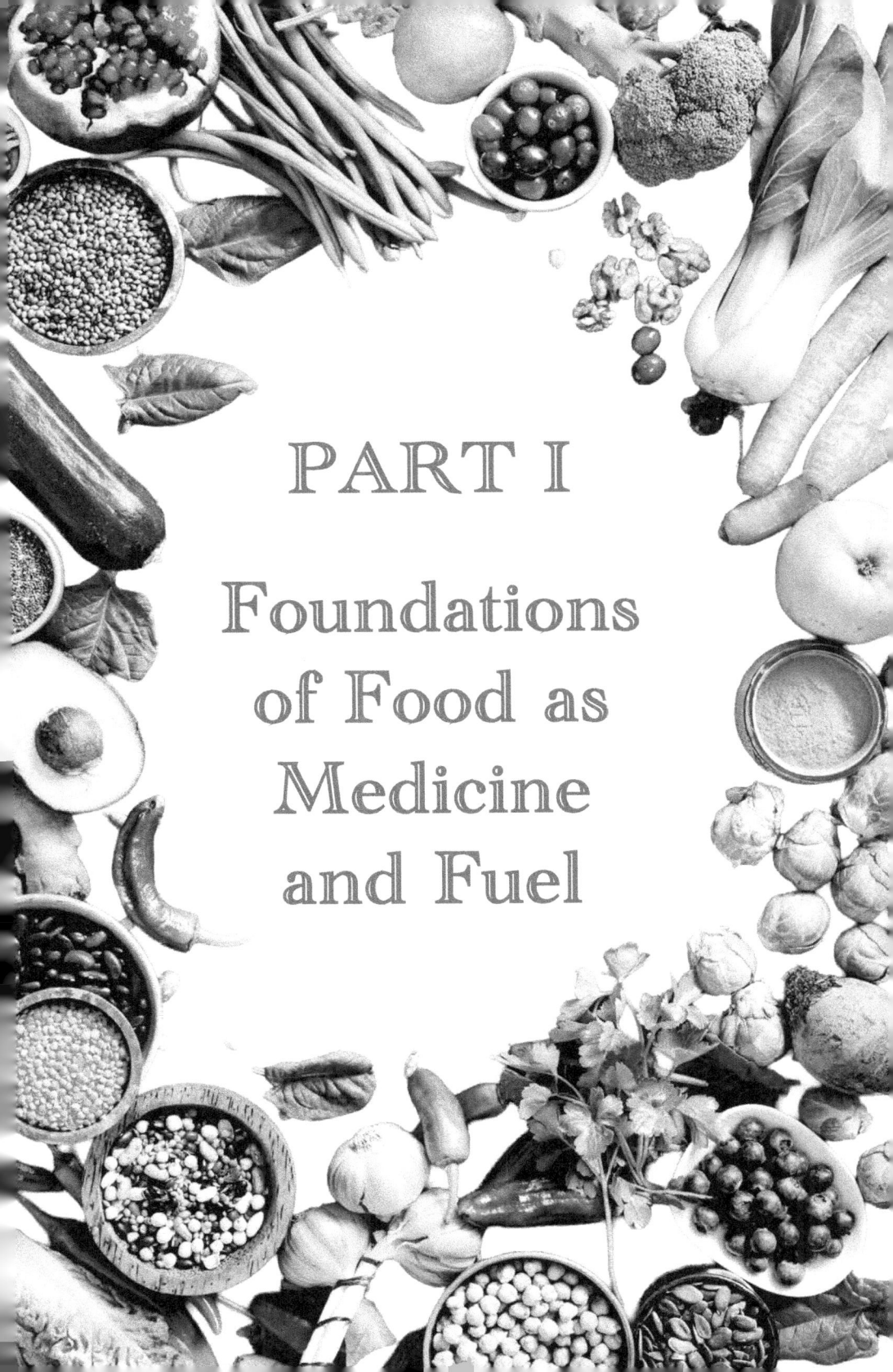

PART I

Foundations of Food as Medicine and Fuel

KEVIN B. DiBacco

CHAPTER 1

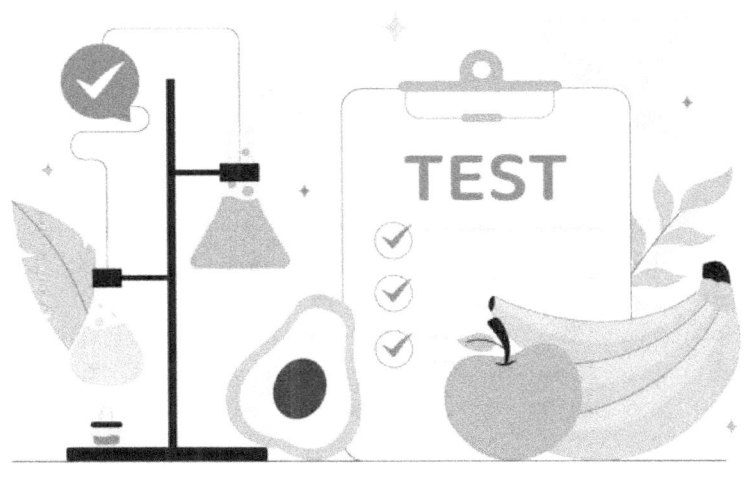

THE SCIENCE BEHIND FOOD AS MEDICINE

Hey there. Ready to dive into the fascinating world of food as medicine? Buckle up because we're about to take a wild ride through history, cutting-edge research, and even your genes. Don't worry, though—I promise to keep things light and fun. No snoozing allowed in this chapter.

A Trip Down Memory Lane
Historical Perspective on Food and Healing

Alright, let's kick things off with a little time travel. Imagine you're in Ancient Greece, hanging out with Hippocrates (yeah, that dude with the oath). He's the one who famously said, "Let food be thy medicine, and medicine be thy food." Pretty ahead of his time, right?

But here's the thing: Hippocrates wasn't alone in thinking food could heal. Cultures all around the world have been using food as medicine for thousands of years.

Take traditional Chinese medicine, for example. These folks were pairing foods with specific health benefits way before it was cool. They believed in the concept of "food energetics," where foods have heating, cooling, or neutral properties that can affect your body's balance. Imagine trying to explain that to your buddy who thinks a balanced diet means equal parts pizza and beer.

Or how about Ayurveda, the traditional medicine system of India? These guys were all about personalizing diet based on your individual constitution, or "dosha." It's like they invented personalized nutrition plans before we even had nutrition labels.

Native American healing traditions also recognized the power of food. They used herbs and plants not just for flavor but for their medicinal properties too. Echinacea, which many of us pop like candy during the cold season, was a staple in their healing practices.

Even in medieval Europe, where medical practices were... let's say "questionable" at times (leeches, anyone?), herbs and foods were often the go-to remedies for various ailments. Garlic for infections, honey for wounds—some of these old-school remedies have stood the test of time and scientific scrutiny.

Now, I know what you're thinking. "That's all ancient history, bro. What does it have to do with me and my protein shake?" Well, hang tight, because we're about to connect the dots between this ancient wisdom and modern science.

MODERN RESEARCH
WHEN SCIENCE CAUGHT UP WITH GRANDMA'S ADVICE

Fast-forward to today, and guess what? Science is finally catching up with what our ancestors seemed to know intuitively. We've got labs, controlled studies, and fancy equipment all backing up the idea that food can be a powerful medicine. Let me throw some mind-blowing facts at you.

HEART HEALTH

Remember when everyone was afraid of eggs? Well, a study in the *American Journal of Clinical Nutrition* showed that eating up to 12 eggs a week didn't increase cardiovascular risk factors in people with pre-diabetes and type 2 diabetes. Take that, egg-haters.

CANCER PREVENTION

A review published in the journal *Cancer Treatment and Research* found that a diet rich in fruits, vegetables, and whole grains could potentially prevent 30–50% of all cancers. That's huge.

BRAIN POWER

Ever heard of the *MIND* diet? It's a combo of the Mediterranean and *DASH* diets, and research in the *Alzheimer's & Dementia Journal* showed it could slow cognitive decline and reduce Alzheimer's risk. Who knew your fork could be a barbell for your brain?

GUT HEALTH

A study in the journal *Cell* showed that switching from a plant-based diet to an animal-based diet changed the microbial composition in the gut in just 24 hours. Talk about fast food.

INFLAMMATION

Research published in the *British Journal of Nutrition* found that people who ate a diet high in fruits, vegetables, nuts, and whole grains had lower levels of inflammatory markers in their blood.

Here's where it gets cool. We're not just talking about preventing disease anymore. We're talking about food as an active player in treating and managing health conditions.

Take the ketogenic diet, for instance. It was originally developed to treat epilepsy in children, and it's been shown to reduce seizures in some cases where medication hasn't worked. That's food doing the job of medicine.

Or how about the role of fiber in managing diabetes? A study in the *New England Journal of Medicine* found that people with type 2 diabetes who increased their fiber intake significantly improved their blood sugar control. That's right—grandma's advice to eat your veggies wasn't about making you "big and strong."

And let's not forget about the gut microbiome—the trillions of bacteria living in your digestive system. This is a hot area of research right now, and for good reason. Studies are showing that the composition of your gut microbiome can influence everything from your mood to your immune system. And guess what influences your gut microbiome? Yep, you guessed it—the food you eat.

A study published in *Nature* showed that a diet high in diverse plant foods led to a more diverse gut microbiome, which is associated with better health outcomes. So next time someone gives you a hard time about your "rabbit food," tell them you're feeding your internal zoo.

Now, I don't know about you, but all this research gets me pumped. It's like we're uncovering superpowers we didn't even know we had, all through the simple act of eating. But hold on to your hats because we're about to go even deeper.

NUTRIGENOMICS
WHEN YOUR DINNER TALKS TO YOUR DNA

Are you ready for some sci-fi-level stuff? Let's talk about nutritionomics. Don't let the fancy term scare you—it's just the study of how food interacts with our genes. Yeah, you heard that right. The burger you had for lunch. It's having a conversation with your DNA right now.

Here's the deal. We used to think our genes were our destiny. You got dealt a certain hand at birth, and that was that. But now we know that while we can't change our genes, we can influence how they express themselves. And one of the biggest influences? You guessed it—food. Let me break it down for you with some examples.

BROCCOLI AND CANCER

There's a compound in broccoli and other cruciferous veggies called sulforaphane. Research has shown that this compound can activate genes that protect against cancer. It's like broccoli is flipping the "off" switch on cancer genes.

OMEGA-3S AND INFLAMMATION

Got some genes that make you more prone to inflammation? Omega-3 fatty acids, found in fatty fish, walnuts, and flaxseeds, can help quiet down those inflammatory genes. It's like giving those overactive genes a chill pill.

RESVERATROL AND AGING

This compound, found in red wine and grapes, has been shown to activate genes associated with longevity. Now, don't go chugging wine by the bottle—but it's cool to think that your glass of pinot might be telling your genes to slow down the aging process.

CURCUMIN AND ALZHEIMER'S

This compound, found in turmeric, has been shown to influence genes involved in the clearance of amyloid plaque in the brain—that's the stuff associated with Alzheimer's disease. Curry night, anyone?

ISOTHIOCYANATES AND DETOXIFICATION

These compounds, found in veggies like Brussels sprouts and cabbage, can activate genes involved in your body's detoxification processes. So next time someone tries to sell you a detox tea, just point them to the produce aisle instead.

Now, before you go thinking you can just eat your way out of any genetic predisposition, let's pump the brakes a bit. Nutrigenomics isn't about completely overriding your genes; it's more about optimizing the hand you've been dealt. Think of it like playing poker. You can't change the cards you're holding, but you can be sure as heck play them better.

And here's where it gets even cooler—this isn't just a one-way street. Just as food can influence our genes, our genetic makeup can influence how we respond to certain foods. This is why some people can drink milk with no problems, while others become best friends with the bathroom after a single latte.

This field of study, called nutrigenetics, is paving the way for truly personalized nutrition. Imagine a future where your diet is tailored not just to your height, weight, and activity level but to your very DNA. We're not there yet, but we're getting closer every day.

PUTTING IT ALL TOGETHER
YOUR FOOD, YOUR MEDICINE CABINET

So, what does all this sciencey stuff mean for you and your dinner plate? Well, it means that every time you sit down to eat, you're not just satisfying your hunger—you're potentially fighting disease, turning genes on and off, and influencing your health in ways we're only beginning to understand.

It's like you've got this incredible pharmacy right in your kitchen. But instead of pills, you've got fruits, veggies, whole grains, lean proteins, and healthy fats. And the best part? The side effects include things like better energy, clearer skin, and jeans that fit just right. Sign me up.

Now, I want to be clear—I'm not saying you should toss out your medications and start treating everything with kale smoothies. Modern medicine is remarkable, and there's absolutely a time and place for conventional treatments. What I am saying is that food can be a powerful tool in your health arsenal, working alongside traditional medicine to help you feel your best.

Remember Sarah, the client I mentioned in the intro who was struggling with fatigue and bloating? When we started focusing on nutrient-dense, whole foods and identified some of her food sensitivities, it was like we'd flipped a switch. Her energy soared, her skin cleared up, and she even lost some weight without really trying. That's the power of using food as medicine.

Or take my experience with inflammation. When I started incorporating more anti-inflammatory foods like fatty fish, berries, and leafy greens while cutting back on processed foods and sugar, my nagging injuries started to heal faster. My recovery time between workouts shortened, and I even noticed my mood improving. It was like I'd discovered a secret weapon—except it wasn't really a secret at all. It was just good, wholesome food.

THE ROAD AHEAD
YOUR JOURNEY TO FOOD AS MEDICINE

So, where do we go from here? Well, my friend, we're just getting started. In the coming chapters, we're going to dive deeper into specific nutrients and how they work in your body. We'll explore how food can be used to manage common health conditions. We'll look at different diet approaches and how to figure out what works best for you.

But for now, I want you to start thinking about food differently. Next time you're planning a meal or reaching for a snack, pause for a moment. Ask yourself, "How is this food going to affect my body? What messages am I sending to my cells, my genes, and my gut microbiome?"

Don't worry, I'm not expecting you to become a nutritional saint overnight. Heck, I still enjoy a good pizza or ice cream cone now and then. The goal isn't perfection; it's progress. It's about making more informed choices, more often. It's about seeing food not just as calories or macros but as a powerful tool for health and healing.

Remember, this is a journey, not a destination. There will be ups and downs, experiments that work and ones that don't. But that's all part of the process. The important thing is that you're taking control of your health, one bite at a time.

So, are you ready to turn your kitchen into your personal pharmacy? Are you excited to become the CEO of your health? Great. We've got a lot of ground to cover, and I can't wait to guide you through it all.

In the next chapter, we're going to break down the building blocks of nutrition—proteins, carbs, fats, vitamins, and minerals. Don't worry, it won't be like your high school chemistry class. We'll keep it fun, practical, and focused on how you can use this knowledge to supercharge your health.

Until then, why not try adding one new "medicinal" food to your diet this week? It's some fatty fish for those omega-3s, or some turmeric for its anti-inflammatory powers. Whatever you choose, pay attention to how it makes you feel. You might just be surprised at the difference a single food can make.

CHAPTER 2

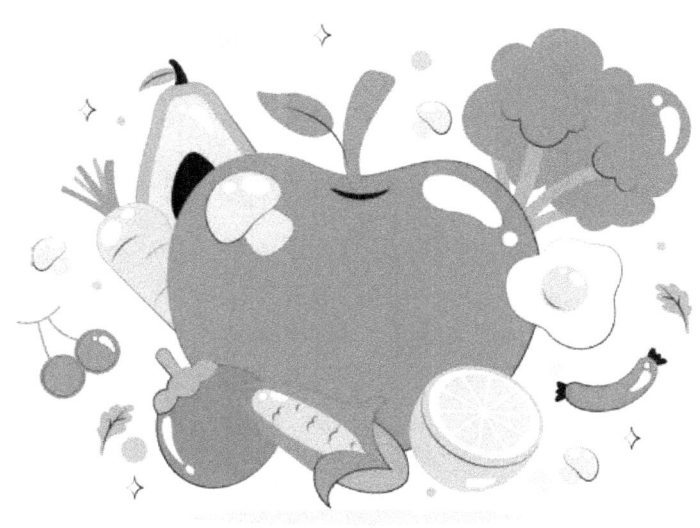

UNDERSTANDING NUTRIENTS

THE BUILDING BLOCKS OF YOUR BODY

What makes your food tick? Don't worry, I promise this won't be like that biology class where you fell asleep with your face in the textbook. We're going to make nutrients fun, I swear.

MACRONUTRIENTS
THE BIG THREE

Let's start with the heavyweights: macronutrients. These are the nutrients you need in large amounts (hence the "macro"). There are three main players in this game: proteins, carbohydrates, and fats. Think of them as the three musketeers of your plate.

PROTEINS: THE BODY'S BUILDING BLOCKS

Alright, gym rats, this one's for you. Proteins are the superstars of the nutrient world. They're involved in every process in your body, from building muscle to making hormones.

Here's a cool fact: proteins are made up of smaller units called amino acids. There are 20 different amino acids, and your body can make some of them on its own. But there are nine that your body can't make; these are called essential amino acids. You've got to get these from your food.

Now, not all proteins are created equal. Animal sources like meat, fish, eggs, and dairy are considered "complete" proteins because they contain all the essential amino acids. Plant sources are often "incomplete," but don't let that scare you, veggie lovers. You can still get all the amino acids you need by eating a variety of plant proteins throughout the day.

A study published in the *American Journal of Clinical Nutrition* found that spreading protein intake evenly throughout the day was more effective for muscle synthesis than eating most protein at dinner, which is what most Americans do. So, think about including some protein at every meal, not just your post-workout shake.

CARBOHYDRATES: YOUR BODY'S PREFERRED FUEL SOURCE

Ah, carbs. The nutrients everyone loves to hate. But here's the thing: your body, especially your brain, loves carbs. They're your body's preferred source of energy.

Carbs come in two main forms: simple and complex. Simple carbs are found in foods like fruits, milk, and table sugar. They're quickly broken down and can cause a rapid spike in blood sugar. Complex carbs, found in whole grains, legumes, and vegetables, take longer to digest and provide a steadier release of energy.

Here's where it gets interesting: not all carbs affect your blood sugar the same way. This is where the glycemic index (GI) comes in. The GI measures how quickly food raises your blood sugar. Foods with a high GI (like white bread) cause a rapid spike, while low-GI foods (like lentils) cause a more gradual rise.

A study in the journal *Diabetes Care* found that a low-GI diet improved blood sugar control and reduced the risk of cardiovascular disease in people with diabetes. So, next time someone tries to demonize all carbs, you can school them on the importance of choosing the right ones.

FATS: NOT THE VILLAIN THEY WERE ONCE THOUGHT TO BE

Remember when fat was public enemy number one? Well, times have changed, my friend. We now know that certain types of fat are crucial for good health.

Fats play a vital role in hormone production, nutrient absorption, and brain function. They also make food taste good and help you feel full. The key is selecting the right kinds of fat. There are four main types of dietary fats.

MONOUNSATURATED FATS

Monounsaturated fats are found in foods like olive oil, avocados, and nuts. These are the "good" fats that can help lower bad cholesterol levels.

POLYUNSATURATED FATS

These include omega-3 and omega-6 fatty acids, found in fatty fish, walnuts, and flaxseeds. They're essential for brain function and can help reduce inflammation.

SATURATED FATS

Saturated fats are found in animal products and some tropical oils. While not as harmful as once thought, it's still best to consume these in moderation.

TRANS FATS

The real villains of the fat world. These artificial fats are found in many processed foods and have been linked to heart disease. The good news? Many countries are banning trans fats in food products.

A landmark study published in the *New England Journal of Medicine* found that a Mediterranean diet high in olive oil or nuts significantly reduced the risk of major cardiovascular events. So don't be afraid of fat—just choose wisely.

MICRONUTRIENTS
SMALL BUT MIGHTY

Now let's talk about the little guys: micronutrients. These are the vitamins and minerals you need in smaller amounts, but don't let their size fool you—they pack a serious punch when it comes to your health.

VITAMINS: YOUR BODY'S LITTLE HELPERS

Vitamins are organic compounds that your body needs to function properly. There are 13 essential vitamins, each with its own special role.

VITAMIN A

Important for vision, immune function, and skin health.

B VITAMINS (B1, B2, B3, B5, B6, B7, B9, B12)

These play crucial roles in energy production, brain function, and cell metabolism.

VITAMIN C

A powerful antioxidant that supports immune function and skin health.

VITAMIN D

Essential for bone health and immune function. Your body can produce this when exposed to sunlight.

Vitamin E

Another antioxidant that protects your cells from damage.

Vitamin K

Essential for blood clotting and bone health.

Here's a fun fact: A study published in the journal *Neurology* found that people with higher levels of vitamins B, C, D, and E had larger brain volumes and better cognitive function. It's like brain food in the most literal sense.

MINERALS: THE SPARK PLUGS OF YOUR BODY

Minerals are inorganic elements that come from the soil and water and are absorbed by plants or animals. Here are some key players.

Calcium

Not just for strong bones. It's also crucial for muscle function and nerve transmission.

Iron

Essential for carrying oxygen in your blood.

Magnesium

Involved in over 300 enzymatic reactions in your body, including energy production and muscle function.

Zinc

Important for immune function and wound healing.

Selenium

A powerful antioxidant that supports thyroid function.

A study in the *Journal of Nutrition* found that higher magnesium intake was associated with a lower risk of type 2 diabetes. Who knew a humble mineral could be so powerful?

PHYTONUTRIENTS AND ANTIOXIDANTS
NATURE'S DISEASE FIGHTERS

Finally, let's talk about phytonutrients and antioxidants. These are compounds found in plants that aren't essential for keeping you alive but can help prevent disease and keep your body working optimally.

Phytonutrients give fruits and vegetables their vibrant colors and have various health benefits. Here are some examples.

LYCOPENE (found in tomatoes)
May reduce the risk of prostate cancer.
ANTHOCYANINS (found in berries)
Can help improve memory and reduce inflammation.

QUERCETIN (found in apples and onions)
May help reduce the risk of heart disease.

A study published in the *American Journal of Clinical Nutrition* found that a diet rich in plant-based foods was associated with a lower risk of all-cause mortality. It's like eating the rainbow isn't just pretty—it could help you live longer.

Antioxidants are substances that can prevent or slow damage to cells caused by free radicals, unstable molecules that the body produces as a reaction to environmental and other pressures. Some well-known antioxidants include vitamins C and E, beta-carotene, and selenium.

A meta-analysis published in the *European Journal of Nutrition* found that higher intake of dietary antioxidants was associated with a reduced risk of certain types of cancer. It's like your food is your own personal bodyguard, fighting off potential threats.

CHAPTER 3

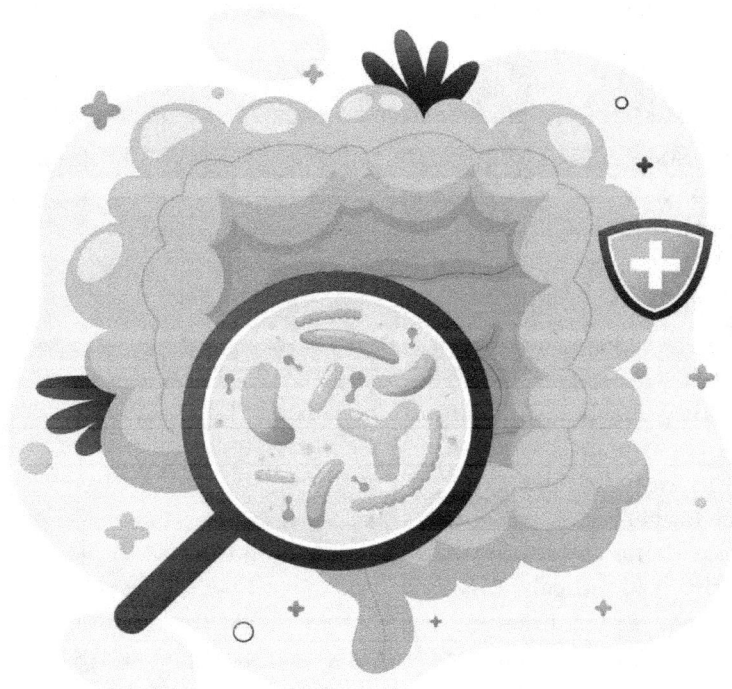

THE GUT-HEALTH CONNECTION

YOUR SECOND BRAIN

One of the hottest topics in health research: your microbiome. That's right, we're going to dive into the world of the trillions of tiny critters living in your gut. Don't worry, they're (mostly) friendly.

THE MICROBIOME
YOUR INTERNAL ECOSYSTEM

Your microbiome is like a bustling city living inside you, with trillions of bacteria, fungi, and other microbes going about their daily business. And just like a city, the diversity of its inhabitants is crucial for everything to run smoothly.

Here's a mind-blowing fact: you have more bacterial cells in your body than human cells. In fact, some scientists estimate that for every one of your cells, there are 1.3 bacterial cells. You're more bacteria than humans. How's that for an identity crisis?

But here's the cool part. Your microbiome isn't just hanging out in your gut doing nothing. It's actively involved in numerous aspects of your health.

DIGESTION
Your gut bacteria help break down foods that your body can't digest on its own, like certain fibers.

NUTRIENT PRODUCTION
Some gut bacteria produce vitamins like B12 and K, which are essential for blood clotting and bone health.

IMMUNE FUNCTION
About 70% of your immune system is in your gut. Your microbiome plays a crucial role in training your immune system to distinguish between friend and foe.

BRAIN FUNCTION
There's a direct line of communication between your gut and your brain, called the gut-brain axis. Your microbiome can influence your mood, behavior, and even cognitive function.

WEIGHT MANAGEMENT

Some studies have found differences in the gut microbiomes of lean and obese individuals, suggesting that your gut bacteria might play a role in weight regulation.

A groundbreaking study published in *Nature* in 2006 found that obese mice had a different composition of gut bacteria compared to lean mice and that this composition could be transferred to germ-free mice, influencing their weight. It's like your gut bacteria are secretly controlling your pants size.

PREBIOTICS AND PROBIOTICS
FEEDING YOUR INTERNAL FRIENDS

Now that we know how important our gut bacteria are, the question is: how do we keep them happy? Enter prebiotics and probiotics, the dynamic duo of gut health.

PREBIOTICS: THE FERTILIZER FOR YOUR GUT GARDEN

Prebiotics are types of dietary fiber that feed the good bacteria in your gut. They're like fertilizer for your internal garden. Some good sources of prebiotics include:

- Garlic

- Onions

- Leeks

- Asparagus

- Bananas

- Oats

A study published in the *British Journal of Nutrition* found that a diet high in prebiotic fiber increased the abundance of beneficial bacteria in the gut and improved calcium absorption. It's like killing two birds with one stone—happy gut, strong bones.

PROBIOTICS: REINFORCEMENTS FOR YOUR BACTERIAL ARMY

Probictics are live bacteria that can provide health benefits when consumed in adequate amounts. They're like reinforcements for your gut's bacterial army. You can find probiotics in fermented foods like:

- Yogurt

- Kefir

- Sauerkraut

- Kimchi

- Kombucha

A meta-analysis published in the *Journal of Clinical Gastroenterology* found that probiotics were effective in treating antibiotic-associated diarrhea. So next time your doctor prescribes antibiotics, you might want to chase them with some yogurt.

LEAKY GUT SYNDROME
WHEN YOUR GUT BARRIER BREAKS DOWN

Now, let's talk about something a bit more serious: leaky gut syndrome. This is a condition where the lining of your intestines becomes more permeable than it should be, allowing partially digested food particles and toxins to "leak" into your bloodstream.

Leaky gut has been associated with a range of health issues, including:

- Autoimmune diseases

- Chronic fatigue syndrome

- Fibromyalgia

☞ Arthritis

☞ Allergies

☞ Acne

While the concept of leaky gut is still controversial in mainstream medicine, research is starting to back it up. A study published in the journal *Gut* found that patients with irritable bowel syndrome had higher intestinal permeability (a.k.a. leakier guts) compared to healthy controls. So, what causes a leaky gut? Several factors can contribute.

POOR DIET
A diet high in sugar and processed foods can lead to inflammation and damage to the gut lining.

CHRONIC STRESS
Stress can weaken your gut barrier and alter the composition of your microbiome.

OVERUSE OF NSAIDS
Non-steroidal anti-inflammatory drugs like ibuprofen can increase intestinal permeability.

EXCESSIVE ALCOHOL CONSUMPTION
Alcohol can directly damage the cells lining your intestines.

NUTRIENT DEFICIENCIES
Certain nutrients like vitamin A, vitamin D, and zinc are crucial for maintaining the integrity of your gut lining.

The good news is that there are ways to support your gut health and potentially heal a leaky gut.

☞ Eat a diverse, whole-food diet rich in fiber.

☞ Include fermented foods in your diet for a probiotic boost.

- ☞ Manage stress through techniques like meditation or yoga.

- ☞ Limit alcohol and NSAID use.

- ☞ Consider supplements like L-glutamine, which can help repair the gut lining.

A study published in the *World Journal of Gastroenterology* found that patients with inflammatory bowel disease who took a glutamine supplement showed improvements in intestinal permeability. It's like giving your gut a repair kit.

WRAPPING IT UP
YOUR NUTRIENTS, YOUR GUT, YOUR HEALTH

So, there you have it, health warriors. We've covered a lot of ground, from the basics of macronutrients to the complexities of your gut microbiome. Here are the key takeaways.

NUTRIENTS ARE THE BUILDING BLOCKS OF YOUR BODY
Make sure you're getting a balance of macronutrients (proteins, carbs, and fats) and micronutrients (vitamins and minerals).

DON'T FORGET ABOUT PHYTONUTRIENTS AND ANTIOXIDANTS
These plant-based compounds can provide powerful health benefits.

YOUR GUT IS LIKE YOUR SECOND BRAIN
Take care of it by eating a diverse diet rich in prebiotics and probiotics.

PAY ATTENTION TO YOUR BODY
Be aware of signs of gut imbalance or leaky gut and take steps to support your gut health.

Remember, every bite you take is an opportunity to nourish your body and support your health. So, choose wisely, but don't stress too much—a little ice cream now and then won't kill you. It's all about balance, my friends.

In the next chapter, we'll dive into how you can use this knowledge to tackle specific health conditions. Get ready to become your own food-as-medicine expert.

Until then, go forth and feed your gut buddies. Your microbiome will thank you.

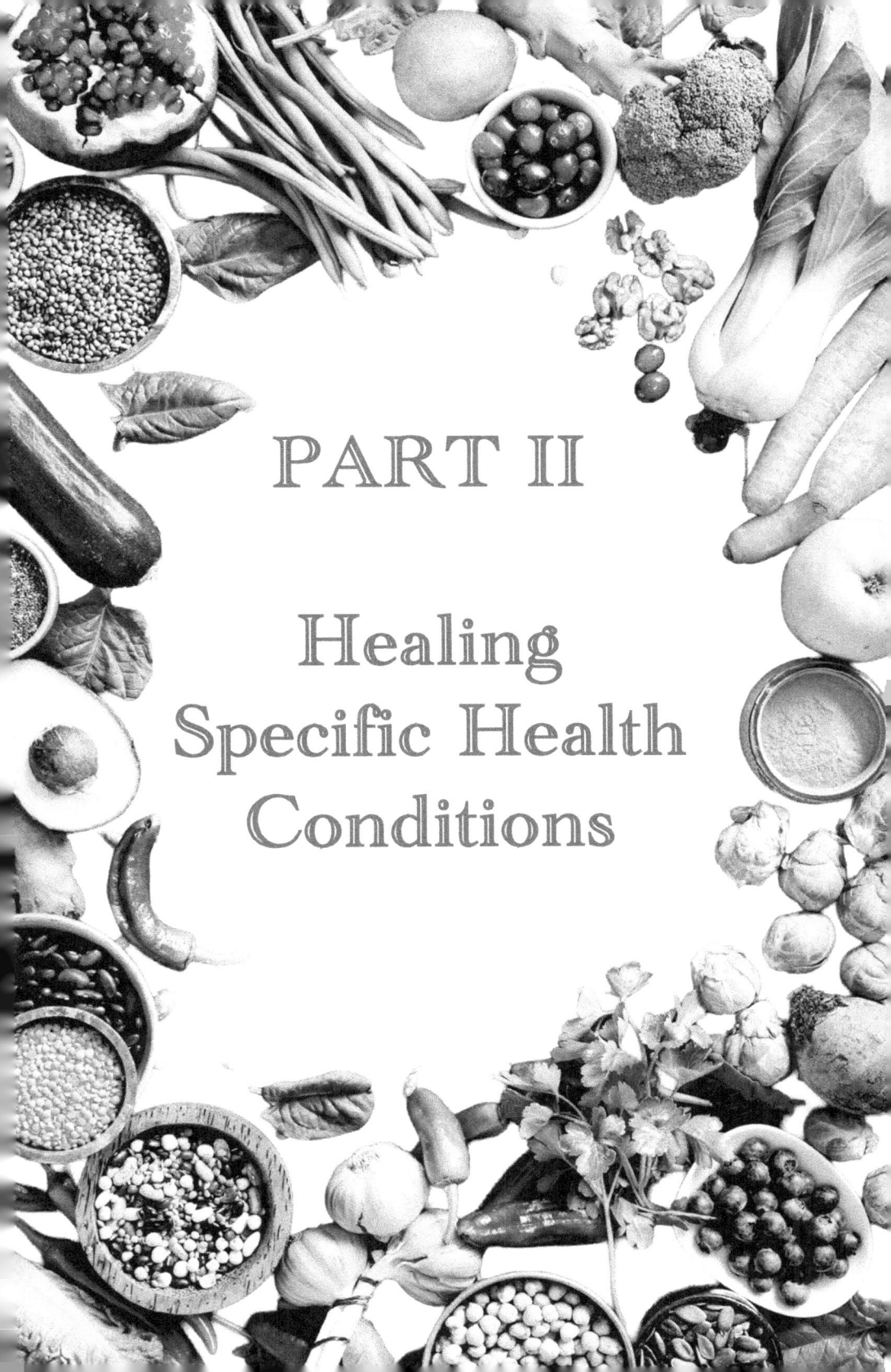

PART II

Healing Specific Health Conditions

CHAPTER 4

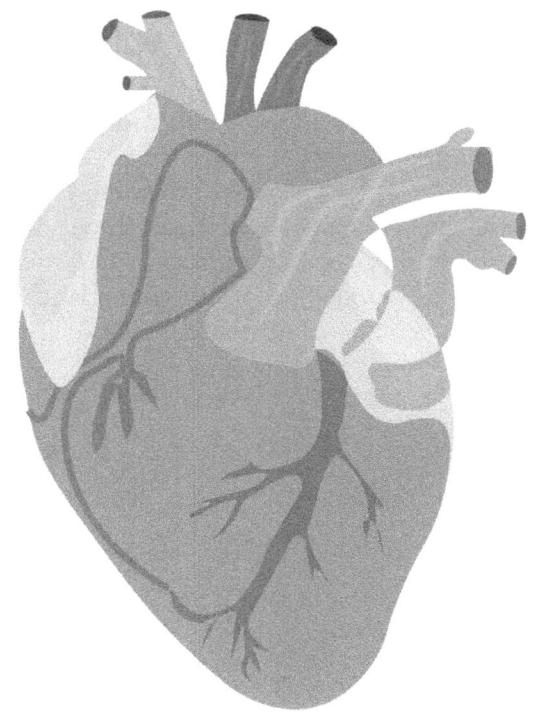

HEART HEALTH

KEEPING YOUR TICKER IN TOP SHAPE

Let's look at that remarkable muscle in your chest that's been working non-stop since before you were born. Yep, we're diving into heart health, and trust me, this is one chapter you would rather not skip. Your heart's been taking care of you your whole life, so let's learn how to return the favor, shall we?

CARDIOVASCULAR DISEASE
THE SILENT KILLER

First things first, let's talk about the boogeyman of the circulatory system: cardiovascular disease (CVD). It's not just one condition, but a whole family of heart and blood vessel problems that can really cramp your style (and your arteries).

Here's a sobering fact to kick us off: According to the World Health Organization, cardiovascular diseases are the number one cause of death globally. In 2019 alone, they took an estimated 17.9 million lives. That's like wiping out the entire population of the Netherlands twice. But don't panic because knowledge is power, and we're about to arm you with plenty of it.

CAUSES AND RISK FACTORS
KNOW YOUR ENEMY

So, what's causing all this cardiac chaos? Well, it's not just one thing (isn't that always the case?). CVD is like a perfect storm of various factors coming together. Let's break it down.

HIGH BLOOD PRESSURE

Imagine your blood vessels are like garden hoses. Now imagine someone's cranked up the water pressure far too high. That's what high blood pressure does to your arteries. Over time, this can damage the lining of your blood vessels, making them more susceptible to plaque buildup.

Fun fact: A study published in *The Lancet* found that reducing salt intake by just 1.25 grams per day could prevent 9 million cases of heart disease and stroke annually. That's a lot of lives saved by putting down the saltshaker.

HIGH CHOLESTEROL

Not all cholesterol is bad (we'll get to that later), but when you've got too much of the wrong kind floating around in your blood, it can start sticking to your artery walls. Over time, this buildup (called plaque) can narrow your arteries, making it harder for blood to flow through.

SMOKING

If your arteries are highways, consider smoking to be throwing nails on the road. It damages your blood vessels, reduces the oxygen in your blood, and increases your risk of blood clots. Not cool, cigarettes. Not cool at all.

DIABETES

High blood sugar can damage your blood vessels and the nerves that control your heart. In fact, adults with diabetes are two to four times more likely to die from heart disease than adults without diabetes, according to the American Heart Association.

OBESITY

Carrying extra weight, especially around your midsection, puts extra strain on your heart and is linked to other risk factors like high blood pressure and diabetes.

LACK OF PHYSICAL ACTIVITY

Your heart is a muscle, and like any muscle, it needs exercise to stay strong. A sedentary lifestyle is like telling your heart to take an extended vacation. Sounds nice, but it's not great for long-term health.

POOR DIET

What you put on your plate has a massive impact on your heart health. A diet high in saturated fats, trans fats, and added sugars can contribute to the buildup of plaque in your arteries.

STRESS

While the exact link between stress and heart disease isn't clear, chronic stress can lead to behaviors that increase your risk, like overeating, smoking, or drinking too much alcohol.

AGE AND FAMILY HISTORY

Some risk factors you can't control. Your risk of heart disease increases as you get older, and if heart disease runs in your family, you might be at higher risk.

Now, before you start feeling like the deck is stacked against you, remember this: many of these risk factors are within your control. And one of the most powerful tools you have for managing them? You guessed it, your diet.

HEART-HEALTHY DIETS
EATING YOUR WAY TO A HEALTHIER HEART

Alright, let's discuss some eating patterns that have been shown to give your heart some serious love.

THE MEDITERRANEAN DIET: SUN, SEA, AND HEART HEALTH

Picture yourself on a beautiful beach in Greece, enjoying fresh fish, olive oil, and a glass of red wine. Sounds like a vacation, right? Well, it turns out this laid-back lifestyle is also great for your heart.

The Mediterranean diet is rich in the following foods.

- Fruits and vegetables

- Whole grains

- legumes and nuts

- Fish and poultry

- Olive oil as the main source of fat

- Moderate amounts of red wine (optional, but who's complaining?)

A landmark study published in the *New England Journal of Medicine* found that participants following a Mediterranean diet supplemented with extra-virgin olive oil or nuts had a significantly lower risk of major cardiovascular events compared to those advised to follow a low-fat diet. Pass the olive oil, please.

THE DASH DIET: DASHING AWAY FROM HIGH BLOOD PRESSURE

DASH stands for Dietary Approaches to Stop Hypertension. It's like the Mediterranean diet's cousin who's really into heart health. The DASH diet focuses on the following foods.

- Fruits and vegetables

- Whole grains

- Lean proteins

- Low-fat dairy

- Limiting sodium, added sugars, and red meat

A study published in the *Archives of Internal Medicine* found that combining the *DASH* diet with sodium reduction led to significant decreases in blood pressure. In some cases, the reduction was as effective as taking blood pressure medication.

THE PORTFOLIO DIET: A HEART-HEALTHY GREATEST HITS

The portfolio diet is like a mixed tape of heart-healthy foods. It includes the following foods.

- Plant proteins (like soy and beans)

- Nuts

- Soluble fiber (found in oats, barley, and eggplant)

☞ Plant sterols (found in vegetable oils and fortified foods)

A study in the *Journal of the American Medical Association* found that people following the Portfolio diet lowered their LDL ("bad") cholesterol by 30% in just four weeks. That's as effective as some cholesterol-lowering medications.

THE PLANT-BASED DIET: POWERED BY PLANTS

While you don't have to go full vegan to reap heart health benefits, increasing your intake of plant-based foods can do wonders for your cardiovascular system. A plant-based diet focuses on these foods.

☞ Fruits and vegetables

☞ Whole grains

☞ Legumes

☞ Nuts and seeds

☞ Limiting or eliminating animal products

A large study published in the *Journal of the American Heart Association* found that a plant-based diet was associated with a lower risk of developing cardiovascular disease and dying from it.

KEY NUTRIENTS FOR HEART HEALTH
YOUR CARDIO ALL-STARS

Now that we've covered some heart-healthy eating patterns, let's zoom in on specific nutrients that are like superheroes for your heart.

OMEGA-3 FATTY ACIDS: THE ANTI-INFLAMMATORY AVENGERS

Found in fatty fish like salmon, mackerel, and sardines, as well as in walnuts and flaxseeds, omega-3s are like a soothing balm for your cardiovascular system. They can help with these issues.

⇪ Lower triglycerides.

⇪ Reduce inflammation.

⇪ Help prevent blood clots.- Potentially lower blood pressure.

A meta-analysis published in *JAMA Internal Medicine* found that consumption of marine omega-3 fatty acids was associated with a lower risk of fatal heart disease.

FIBER: THE CHOLESTEROL BUSTER

Fiber, especially soluble fiber, is like a street sweeper for your arteries. It can help lower your LDL cholesterol by binding to cholesterol particles in your digestive system and moving them out of your body. Here are some great sources of fiber!

⇪ Oats

⇪ Barley

⇪ Beans

⇪ Apples

⇪ Citrus fruits

A study in the *American Journal of Clinical Nutrition* found that for every 10 grams of fiber you add to your daily diet, your risk of death from heart disease declines by 17%. Now that's what I call functional food.

POTASSIUM: THE PRESSURE RELIEVER

Potassium helps your body get rid of excess sodium, which can help lower your blood pressure. It's like a bouncer, kicking out the troublemakers (sodium) that are causing a ruckus in your blood vessels. Find potassium in these great tasting foods!

- Bananas

- Sweet potatoes

- Spinach

- Beans

- Avocados

A meta-analysis published in the Journal of the American College of Cardiology found that increased potassium intake was associated with lower blood pressure in people with hypertension.

ANTIOXIDANTS: THE FREE RADICAL FIGHTERS

Antioxidants, like vitamins C and E, beta-carotene, and lycopene, help protect your cells from damage caused by free radicals. They're like your body's personal bodyguards. You can find antioxidants in these types of food.

- Berries

- Dark leafy greens

- Tomatoes

- Nuts

- Dark chocolate (yes, you read that right.)

A study in the *European Journal of Preventive Cardiology* found that a diet high in antioxidant-rich foods was associated with a lower risk of heart attack in women.

PLANT STEROLS AND STANOLS: THE CHOLESTEROL IMPOSTERS

These compounds, found naturally in plants, are structurally like cholesterol. They can help block the absorption of cholesterol in your gut, potentially lowering your LDL levels. You can find them in these foods.

- ☞ Vegetable oils

- ☞ Nuts

- ☞ Seeds

- ☞ Fortified foods

A review published in the *Journal of the American Dietetic Association* found that consuming 2 grams of plant sterols or stanols per day can lower LDL cholesterol by 10%.

MAGNESIUM: THE RHYTHM KEEPER

Magnesium plays a crucial role in maintaining a normal heart rhythm and healthy blood pressure. It's like the conductor of your heart's orchestra. Here is a list of foods containing magnesium.

- ☞ Spinach

- ☞ Almonds

- ☞ Black beans

- ☞ Avocado

- ☞ Whole grains

A meta-analysis in the *American Journal of Clinical Nutrition* found that higher magnesium intake was associated with a lower risk of cardiovascular disease.

PUTTING IT ALL TOGETHER
YOUR HEART-HEALTHY GAME PLAN

Alright, heart heroes, let's recap and put together a game plan for keeping your ticker in top shape.

FOCUS on a plant-based diet rich in fruits, vegetables, whole grains, and lean proteins.

INCLUDE fatty fish in your diet 2–3 times a week for those omega-3s.

SNACK on nuts and seeds for a heart-healthy boost.

USE olive oil as your primary cooking fat.

LIMIT saturated fats, trans fats, added sugars, and excess sodium.

STAY ACTIVE and aim for at least 150 minutes of moderate-intensity exercise per week.

MANAGE STRESS through techniques like meditation, yoga, or deep breathing exercises.

If you smoke, WORK ON QUITTING. Your heart (and the rest of your body) will thank you.

KEEP TABS on your blood pressure, cholesterol, and blood sugar levels.

REMEMBER, small changes can add up to big results over time.

A WORD OF
CAUTION

While food can be incredibly powerful in promoting heart health, it's not a substitute for medical care. If you have existing heart issues or are at high risk for cardiovascular disease, it's crucial to work with your healthcare provider. They can help you develop a personalized plan that may include both dietary changes and medication if necessary.

Remember, your heart's been beating for you non-stop since before you were born. It's time we showed it some love back. By making heart-healthy food choices, you're not just reducing your risk of cardiovascular disease, you're investing in a healthier, happier future.

So, are you ready to become a heart health hero? Great. Let's get out there and show our hearts some love, one delicious, nutritious bite at a time. Your future self (and your heart) will thank you.

CHAPTER 5

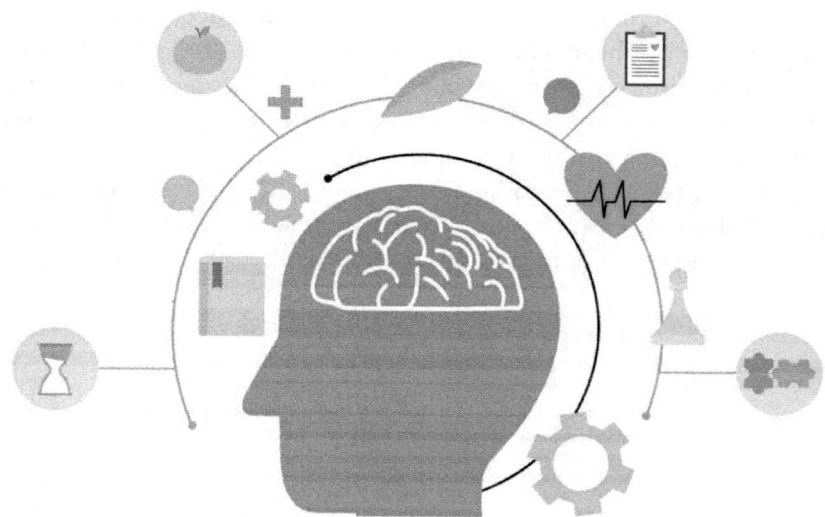

BRAIN HEALTH AND COGNITIVE FUNCTION

FOOD FOR THOUGHT

The brain. It's time to feed that beautiful, complex organ sitting between your ears. Your brain might only weigh about 3 pounds (1.36 kg), but it uses a whopping 20% of your body's energy. Talk about an energy hog. But hey, it's working hard to keep you thinking, feeling, and functioning, so let's make sure we're giving it the premium fuel it deserves.

NUTRITION FOR MEMORY AND FOCUS
FEEDING YOUR MENTAL MUSCLES

Just like your biceps need protein to grow, your brain needs specific nutrients to stay sharp. Let's break down some key players in the game of mental fitness.

OMEGA-3 FATTY ACIDS: THE BRAIN'S BFF

Omega-3s, particularly DHA (docosahexaenoic acid), are like superfoods for your neurons. They're crucial for brain structure and function. Here's the scoop.

SOURCES
Fatty fish (salmon, mackerel, sardines), walnuts, flaxseeds, chia seeds.

BENEFITS
Improved memory, better focus, reduced risk of cognitive decline.

A study published in the journal *Neurology* found that people with higher levels of omega-3s had larger brain volumes and performed better on tests of memory and abstract thinking. It's like giving your brain a growth spurt.

B VITAMINS: THE ENERGY BOOSTERS

B vitamins, especially B6, B12, and folate, are like the spark plugs for your brain cells. They help produce energy and neurotransmitters.

SOURCES
Whole grains, leafy greens, eggs, lean meats.

BENEFITS

Enhanced cognitive function, improved mood, potentially reduced risk of cognitive decline.

Research published in the *American Journal of Clinical Nutrition* showed that older adults with higher blood levels of B vitamins had slower rates of brain atrophy. It's like hitting the brakes on brain aging.

ANTIOXIDANTS: THE BRAIN'S BODYGUARDS

Antioxidants like vitamins C and E, beta-carotene, and flavonoids protect your brain cells from oxidative stress. They're like bouncers, keeping the troublemakers (free radicals) out of your brain's exclusive club.

SOURCES

Berries, dark chocolate, nuts, colorful fruits, and vegetables.

BENEFITS

Improved memory, enhanced cognitive function, and potential protection against neurodegenerative diseases.

A study in the *Annals of Neurology* found that women who consumed more berries had slower rates of cognitive decline as they aged. Berries for the win.

CHOLINE: THE MEMORY MAESTRO

Choline is a precursor to acetylcholine, a neurotransmitter crucial for memory and learning. It's like the conductor of your brain's memory orchestra.

SOURCES

Eggs, liver, soybeans, and peanuts.

BENEFITS

Improved memory and cognitive function.

Research in the *American Journal of Clinical Nutrition* showed that higher choline intake was associated with better cognitive performance in middle-aged and older adults. Time to get cracking on those eggs.

CAFFEINE: THE FOCUS ENHANCER

While not a nutrient per se, caffeine deserves a mention for its cognitive-boosting effects. It's like a temporary turboboost for your brain.

SOURCES

Coffee, tea, and dark chocolate.

BENEFITS

Improved alertness, enhanced focus, potentially reduced risk of cognitive decline.

A study in *Nature Neuroscience* found that caffeine can enhance certain memories for up to 24 hours after consumption. Just remember, moderation is key—too much caffeine can lead to jitters and sleep problems.

DIETARY APPROACHES TO PREVENT NEURODEGENERATIVE DISEASES
NOURISHING YOUR NEURONS

Now that we've covered some brain-boosting nutrients, let's look at some dietary patterns that have been associated with reduced risk of neurodegenerative diseases like Alzheimer's and Parkinson's.

THE MEDITERRANEAN DIET
SUN, SEA, AND BRAIN HEALTH

We've talked about this diet before for heart health, but it's a superstar for brain health too. Here's why.

- Rich in fruits, vegetables, whole grains, and healthy fats.

- Emphasizes fish and limits red meat.

- Includes moderate consumption of red wine (hello, resveratrol).

A study published in *Neurology* found that older adults who followed a Mediterranean diet had a 35% lower risk of cognitive impairment. That's some serious food for thought.

THE MIND DIET
MEDITERRANEAN DIET'S BRAIN-BOOSTING COUSIN

MIND stands for the combination of the Mediterranean and DASH (Intervention for Neurodegenerative Delay) diets. It's like a greatest hits album of brain-healthy foods. Key components include the following.

- Green leafy vegetables

- Other vegetables

- Nuts

- Berries

- Beans

- Whole grains

- Fish

- Poultry

- Olive oil

- Wine (in moderation)

Research published in *Alzheimer's & Dementia* showed that strict adherence to the MIND diet was associated with a 53% reduced rate of Alzheimer's disease. Now that's what I call smart eating.

KETOGENIC DIET
FUELING YOUR BRAIN WITH FAT

The ketogenic diet, high in fats and low in carbs, has shown promise in neurological health. Here's the deal.

- ☞ Forces your body to use ketones (derived from fat) for fuel instead of glucose.

- ☞ May provide an alternative energy source for brain cells.

- ☞ Could potentially reduce inflammation and oxidative stress in the brain.

A study in *Neurobiology of Aging* found that older adults at risk for Alzheimer's showed improved memory performance after following a ketogenic diet. However, more research is needed, and this diet isn't suitable for everyone, so always consult a healthcare professional before making drastic dietary changes.

INTERMITTENT FASTING
GIVING YOUR BRAIN A BREAK

Intermittent fasting isn't weight loss; it might have brain-boosting benefits too. Here's how. Intermittent fasting may promote the growth of new nerve cells; could enhance the brain's ability to adapt to new situations (neuroplasticity); and might reduce inflammation and oxidative stress. Research in the journal *Cell Metabolism* suggests that intermittent fasting could delay the onset of Alzheimer's and Parkinson's disease in animal models. While more human studies are needed, it's an intriguing area of research.

THE GUT-BRAIN AXIS
YOUR SECOND BRAIN

Alright, here's where things get interesting. Your gut and your brain are in constant communication, like two best friends who can't stop texting each other. This information superhighway is called the gut-brain axis, and it's changing how we think about brain health. Here are some mind-blowing facts about the gut-brain connection.

- ☞ Your gut produces about 95% of your body's serotonin, a neurotransmitter that regulates mood, sleep, and appetite. That's right, your gut feelings are real.

- ☞ The bacteria in your gut can influence your brain chemistry and mental health. A study in gastroenterology found that people with depression had different gut bacteria compared to non-depressed individuals.

- ☞ Stress can alter the composition of your gut bacteria, potentially leading to digestive issues and mood changes. It's a two-way street.

So, how can we nurture this gut-brain relationship? Here are some strategies.

PROBIOTICS

These beneficial bacteria can support both gut and brain health. A study in *Frontiers in Aging Neuroscience* found that probiotic supplementation improved cognitive function in Alzheimer's patients.

PREBIOTICS

These fibers feed your good gut bacteria. Research in psychopharmacology indicated that prebiotic intake reduced stress hormone levels in healthy adults.

FERMENTED FOODS

Things like yogurt, kefir, and sauerkraut can provide both prebiotics and probiotics. A study in *Clinical Psychopharmacology and Neuroscience* found that fermented food consumption was associated with lower social anxiety in young adults.

DIVERSITY IN PLANT FOODS

The more diverse your diet, the more diverse (and healthier) your gut microbiome. A study in the *American Journal of Clinical Nutrition* found that a diet high in different plant foods was associated with greater microbial diversity.

Remember, a happy gut often means a happy brain.

CHAPTER 6

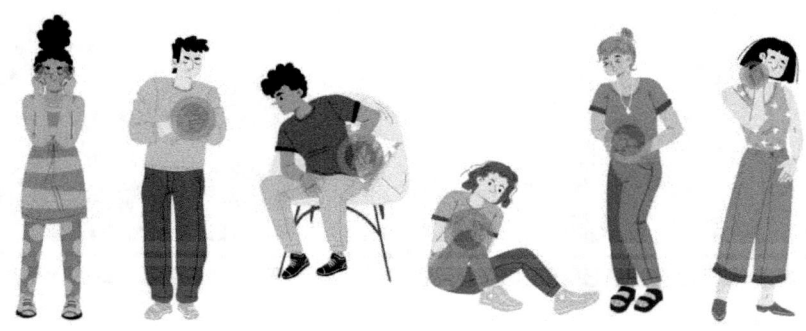

MANAGING CHRONIC PAIN THROUGH DIET

EATING AWAY AT PAIN

Pain sufferers, did you know what's on your plate could help manage that persistent ache? Chronic pain is like that annoying neighbor who won't stop playing loud music at 2 AM. It's disruptive, frustrating, and can seriously impact your quality of life. But what if I told you that your fork could be a powerful weapon in this fight? Let's dig in.

INFLAMMATORY FOODS TO AVOID
THE PAIN PROMOTERS

First things first—let's talk about the troublemakers. These are foods that can increase inflammation in your body, potentially exacerbating pain. Here's the lineup of usual suspects.

ADDED SUGARS: THE SWEET SABOTEURS

Sugar isn't just bad for your waistline—it can be a pain in the, well, everything. Here's why.

- Triggers the release of inflammatory messengers called cytokines.

- Can lead to increased inflammation and pain sensitivity.

A study published in the *Journal of Pain* found that reducing sugar intake led to decreased pain sensitivity in as little as 9 days. Talk about a sweet deal.

TRANS FATS: THE ARTIFICIAL AGITATORS

These artificial fats are like little fire starters in your body, igniting inflammation wherever they go.

- Found in many processed and fried foods.

- Can increase systemic inflammation.

Research in the *Journal of Nutrition* showed that higher intake of trans fats was associated with increased markers of systemic inflammation. Time to say goodbye to those donuts.

REFINED CARBOHYDRATES: THE WHITE MENACE

White bread, pasta, and other refined carbs might taste delicious, but they're not doing your pain levels any favors.

- ✐ Quickly convert to sugar in your body, leading to insulin spikes.

- ✐ Can promote inflammation.

A study in the *American Journal of Clinical Nutrition* found that a diet high in refined carbohydrates was associated with increased levels of inflammatory markers. It's time to embrace those whole grains.

OMEGA-6 FATTY ACIDS (IN EXCESS): TOO MUCH OF A GOOD THING

While we need some omega-6 fats, most of us get far too much, throwing off our omega-3 to omega-6 ratio.

- ✐ Found in many vegetable oils and processed foods.

- ✐ Can promote inflammation when consumed in excess.

Research in biomedicine and pharmacotherapy suggests that a high omega-6 to omega-3 ratio can contribute to the development of various chronic diseases, including those involving pain.

ALCOHOL: THE INFLAMMATORY INTOXICANT

While a glass of wine might help you relax, too much alcohol can amp up inflammation.

- ✐ Can disrupt gut bacteria balance.

- ✐ May increase intestinal permeability, leading to more inflammation.

A study in *Alcohol Research: Current Reviews* found that chronic alcohol consumption can lead to increased systemic inflammation. Moderation is key, folks.

ANTI-INFLAMMATORY DIETS AND NUTRIENTS
YOUR PAIN-FIGHTING ARSENAL

Now that we know what to avoid, let's talk about what to embrace. These foods and nutrients are like your body's own anti-inflammatory SWAT team.

MEDITERRANEAN DIET: THE GOLD STANDARD
We've sung its praises for heart and brain health, and guess what? It's great for managing inflammation too.

- Rich in fruits, vegetables, whole grains, lean proteins, and healthy fats.

- Low in processed foods and added sugars.

A study in rheumatology found that adhering to a Mediterranean diet was associated with reduced pain and increased physical function in people with osteoarthritis. Olive oil, anyone?

OMEGA-3 FATTY ACIDS: THE INFLAMMATION FIGHTERS
These healthy fats are like fire extinguishers for inflammation.

- Found in fatty fish, walnuts, flaxseeds, and chia seeds.

- Can help reduce inflammation and pain.

Research published in *Pain* showed that omega-3 supplementation reduced pain and improved function in people with rheumatoid arthritis. Fish for dinner, anyone?

TURMERIC: THE GOLDEN SPICE
Curcumin, the active compound in turmeric, is a powerful anti-inflammatory.

- Can inhibit inflammatory pathways in the body.

- May help reduce pain in conditions like arthritis.

A study in the *Journal of Medicinal Food* found that turmeric extract reduced pain and improved function in people with knee osteoarthritis. Time to spice up your life.

GINGER: THE ZESTY PAIN RELIEVER

This spicy root isn't just for settling upset stomachs. It's a potent anti-inflammatory too.

- ☞ Contains compounds that inhibit inflammation.

- ☞ May help reduce muscle pain and soreness.

Research in arthritis research and therapy showed that ginger supplementation reduced pain and inflammation in people with osteoarthritis. Ginger tea, anyone?

ANTIOXIDANT-RICH FOODS: THE FREE RADICAL SCAVENGERS

Berries, leafy greens, and other colorful fruits and vegetables are packed with antioxidants that can help combat inflammation.

- ☞ Help neutralize harmful free radicals.

- ☞ May reduce oxidative stress and inflammation.

A study in antioxidants found that a diet rich in fruits and vegetables was associated with lower levels of inflammatory markers. Eat the rainbow, folks.

PROBIOTICS: THE GUT-INFLAMMATION CONNECTION

Remember our talk about the gut-brain axis? Well, it turns out a healthy gut can also help manage inflammation and pain.

- ☞ Can help balance gut bacteria.

- ☞ May reduce systemic inflammation.

Research in the *Pain Physician* journal found that probiotic supplementation reduced pain and improved quality of life in people with chronic pain conditions. Your gut will thank you.

CASE STUDIES AND RESEARCH
REAL-WORLD PAIN MANAGEMENT

Let's look at some real-world examples of how diet can impact chronic pain.

FIBROMYALGIA AND THE LOW-FODMAP DIET
FODMAPs are types of carbohydrates that can be poorly absorbed in the gut, potentially leading to digestive issues and inflammation.

A study published in *Clinical and Experimental Rheumatology* found that a low-FODMAP diet reduced pain scores in people with fibromyalgia. Participants reported a 24–31% reduction in pain severity after following the diet for 8 weeks. That's some serious food power.

RHEUMATOID ARTHRITIS AND VEGAN DIET
A plant-based diet might help cool the flames of inflammation in rheumatoid arthritis.

Research in arthritis research and therapy showed that a vegan diet rich in probiotics significantly decreased pain and improved functional status in patients with rheumatoid arthritis. After just 3 months, participants reported a 53% decrease in joint pain.

MIGRAINE AND KETOGENIC DIET
The high-fat, low-carb ketogenic diet might help put the brakes on migraine pain.

A study in the *European Journal of Neurology* found that a ketogenic diet reduced the frequency and duration of migraine attacks. After one month, 90% of participants reported fewer attacks, and 50% experienced a reduction in attack frequency of more than 50%. Now that's what I call a headache remedy.

BACK PAIN AND AN ANTI-INFLAMMATORY DIET
Chronic low back pain is a common complaint, but diet might help provide some relief.

Research in pain medicine indicated that an anti-inflammatory diet intervention reduced pain and improved quality of life in people with chronic low back pain. After 16 weeks, participants reported a 36% reduction in pain intensity. That's nothing to slouch about.

OSTEOARTHRITIS AND MEDITERRANEAN DIET

The Mediterranean diet strikes again, this time taking on osteoarthritis. A study in *Clinical Nutrition* found that greater adherence to a Mediterranean diet was associated with a lower prevalence of knee osteoarthritis. Participants with the highest adherence to the diet had a 50% lower risk of knee osteoarthritis compared to those with the lowest adherence. Olive oil for the win.

PUTTING IT ALL TOGETHER
YOUR PAIN MANAGEMENT PLATE

So, what does all this mean for you and your chronic pain? Here's a simple game plan to get you started.

OUT WITH THE BAD

Start by gradually reducing your intake of inflammatory foods. Small changes can add up to big results over time.

IN WITH THE GOOD

Focus on incorporating more anti-inflammatory foods into your diet. Think colorful fruits and veggies, fatty fish, nuts, seeds, and spices like turmeric and ginger.

EXPERIENCE

Everyone's body is different. What works for one person might not work for another. Keep a food diary to track how different foods affect your pain levels.

BE PATIENT

Dietary changes don't work overnight. Give it time—at least a few weeks—before deciding if a particular approach is working for you.

STAY HYDRATED

Drinking plenty of water can help flush out inflammatory toxins from your body.

REMEMBER THE BASICS

While diet is important, don't neglect other aspects of pain management like exercise, stress reduction, and getting enough sleep.

WORK WITH PROFESSIONALS

Always consult your healthcare provider before making significant changes to your diet, especially if you're managing a chronic condition.

Remember, food isn't a magic cure-all for chronic pain, but it can be a powerful tool in your pain management toolkit. By making informed choices about what you put on your plate, you're taking an active role in managing your pain and improving your health.

So, pain warriors, are you ready to wage war on inflammation with your fork and knife? Great. Let's dive deeper into some strategies and considerations for using diet to manage chronic pain.

THE ROLE OF WEIGHT MANAGEMENT IN PAIN REDUCTION

One aspect we haven't touched on yet is the connection between excess weight and chronic pain, particularly in conditions like osteoarthritis. Carrying extra pounds puts additional stress on your joints, which can exacerbate pain. But here's some good news. A study published in *Arthritis Care & Research* found that overweight and obese adults with knee osteoarthritis who lost at least 10% of their body weight experienced significant improvements in pain, function, and quality of life. The best part? The more weight they lost, the greater the benefits.

So, if you're carrying extra weight, focusing on a healthy, balanced diet that promotes gradual weight loss could be a double whammy for pain management, reducing inflammation and decreasing physical stress on your joints.

The importance of consistency when it comes to using diet to manage chronic pain, consistency is key. It's not about perfect adherence to a specific diet 100% of the time, but rather about making sustainable changes that you can stick with long-term.

A study in the journal *Pain* found that patients with chronic pain who consistently followed an anti-inflammatory diet reported significant reductions in pain intensity and improved quality of life after just eight weeks. However, these benefits were only maintained in those who continued to follow the diet.

Remember, it's not about perfection; it's about progress. Small, consistent changes can add up to big results over time.

Mindful Eating and Chronic Pain

Here's an interesting twist. The way you eat might be just as important as what you eat when it comes to managing chronic pain. Mindful eating, which involves paying full attention to the experience of eating and drinking, has been shown to have potential benefits for chronic pain management.

A study published in the *Journal of Behavioral Medicine* found that a mindful eating intervention led to significant reductions in pain-related distress and improvements in quality of life in individuals with chronic pain conditions.

So, next time you sit down for a meal, try to really focus on the experience. Notice the colors, smells, textures, and flavors of your food. This practice not only helps you enjoy your food more but might also contribute to pain management.

The Role of Timing in Pain Management

When you eat, it might also play a role in pain management. Some research suggests that intermittent fasting or time-restricted eating might have anti-inflammatory effects that could benefit those with chronic pain.

A study in *Cell Reports* found that time-restricted feeding (limiting food intake to a 6-hour period daily) reduced inflammation and improved gut health in mice. While more research is needed in humans, this suggests that when we eat might be another tool in our pain management arsenal.

Supplements for Pain Management

While whole foods should be the foundation of your anti-inflammatory diet, certain supplements might provide additional support for pain management. Here are a few that have shown promise.

Fish Oil

Rich in omega-3 fatty acids, fish oil has potent anti-inflammatory effects. A meta-analysis published in *Pain Physician* found that fish oil supplementation significantly reduced joint pain intensity in patients with rheumatoid arthritis and other inflammatory joint diseases.

VITAMIN D

Low levels of vitamin D have been associated with increased pain sensitivity. A study in the *Clinical Journal of Pain* found that vitamin D supplementation reduced pain in adults with vitamin D deficiency.

GLUCOSAMINE AND CHONDROITIN

These supplements are popular for joint health. While results are mixed, some studies have found benefits. For instance, a study in the *New England Journal of Medicine* found that the combination of glucosamine and chondroitin provided significant pain relief for people with moderate-to-severe knee osteoarthritis.

Remember, always consult your healthcare provider before starting any new supplement regimen, especially if you're taking other medications.

THE EMOTIONAL SIDE OF EATING AND PAIN

Let's not forget the complex relationship between emotions, eating, and pain. Chronic pain can be incredibly stressful, and many people turn to food for comfort. While this is completely understandable, emotional eating can sometimes lead to choices that may increase inflammation and pain eventually.

A study in the *Journal of Pain Research* found that emotional eating was associated with increased pain intensity and decreased quality of life in individuals with chronic pain. The researchers suggested that addressing emotional eating could be an important part of comprehensive pain management.

If you find yourself turning to food for emotional reasons, consider working with a mental health professional or a registered dietitian who specializes in emotional eating. They can help you develop healthier coping strategies and expand your relationship with food.

Bringing It All Together
Your Personalized Pain Management Plan

As we wrap up our exploration of diet and chronic pain, remember that there's no one-size-fits-all approach. Your journey to managing pain through diet will be as unique as you are. Here are some steps to help you create your personalized plan.

Start with a Food Diary

For a week or two, write down everything you eat and drink, along with your pain levels. This can help you identify potential trigger foods or eating patterns that might be exacerbating your pain.

Gradually Introduce Changes

Instead of overhauling your entire diet overnight, start with small, manageable changes. Maybe swap out refined grains for whole grains or add an extra serving of vegetables to your daily meals.

Experiment with Different Anti-Inflammatory Foods

Try incorporating foods like fatty fish, berries, leafy greens, nuts, and spices like turmeric and ginger into your meals. Pay attention to how you feel after eating these foods.

Consider Consulting a Professional

A registered dietitian or a healthcare provider with expertise in nutrition can help you create a personalized eating plan that considers your specific health needs and food preferences.

Be Patient and Persistent

Remember, dietary changes take time to show effects. Give your new eating habits at least a few weeks before evaluating their impact on your pain levels.

DON'T NEGLECT OTHER ASPECTS OF PAIN MANAGEMENT

While diet can be a powerful tool, it's most effective when used as part of a comprehensive pain management strategy that includes physical activity, stress management, and appropriate medical care.

CLOSING THOUGHTS ON BRAIN HEALTH AND PAIN MANAGEMENT

As we conclude our deep dive into brain health and chronic pain management, it's worth noting the intricate connections between these two areas. Chronic pain can have significant impacts on cognitive function and mental health, and conversely, cognitive strategies can play a role in pain management.

A study published in the journal *Pain* found that chronic pain was associated with accelerated cognitive decline in older adults. This underscores the importance of a holistic approach to health that addresses both physical pain and cognitive function.

The good news is that many of the dietary strategies we've discussed for pain management—like following a Mediterranean-style diet rich in fruits, vegetables, whole grains, and healthy fats—are also beneficial for brain health. It's a beautiful example of how taking care of one aspect of your health often has ripple effects that benefit your entire wellbeing.

Remember, your brain and body are not separate entities but parts of an interconnected whole. By nourishing your body with anti-inflammatory foods, you're not just managing pain; you're also supporting your brain health, mood, and quality of life.

As you embark on this journey of using food as medicine for pain management and brain health, be kind to yourself. Celebrate small victories, be patient with setbacks, and remember that every healthy choice you make is a step in the right direction.

Here's to your health, happiness, and a future with less pain and more vitality. You've got this.

CHAPTER 7

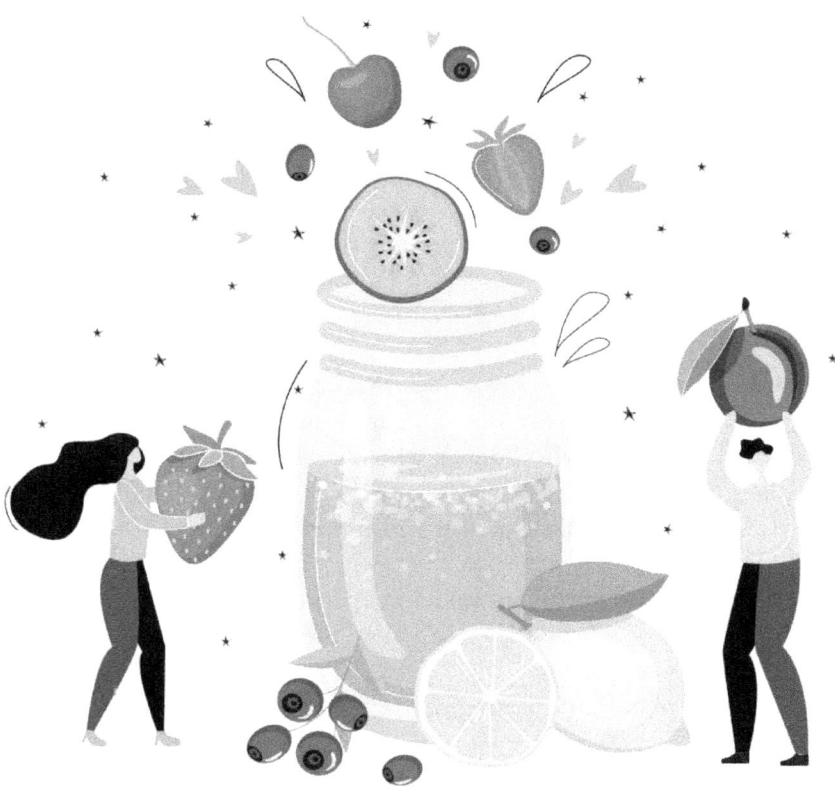

BOOSTING IMMUNITY AND FEEDING YOUR BODY'S DEFENSE SYSTEM

Now the immunity warriors. Your body's very own superhero team, your immune system. This incredible network of cells, tissues, and organs works tirelessly to protect you from invaders like bacteria, viruses, and other nasty things that want to crash your body's party. And guess what? The fuel you provide this superhero team can make a huge difference in how well they do their job. So, let's dive into how you can eat your way to a stronger immune system.

NUTRIENTS ESSENTIAL FOR IMMUNE FUNCTION
THE SUPERHERO FUEL

Just like any good superhero needs the right gear, your immune system needs specific nutrients to function at its best. Let's break down some key players.

VITAMIN C: THE IMMUNE SYSTEM'S FAVORITE SIDEKICK
Vitamin C is like the Robin to your immune system's Batman, always there to lend a helping hand. Here's why it's so crucial.

- It stimulates the production and function of white blood cells.

- Acts as a powerful antioxidant, protecting immune cells from damage.

- It helps maintain the integrity of your skin, your body's first line of defense.

A study published in *Nutrients* found that vitamin C deficiency was associated with impaired immunity and higher susceptibility to infections. Time to stock up on those citrus fruits.

SOURCES OF VITAMIN C

- Strawberries

- Bell peppers

- Broccoli

☞ Potatoes

VITAMIN D: THE SUNSHINE VITAMIN

Vitamin D isn't just for strong bones; it's a key player in immune function too. Here's the scoop.

☞ Activates T cells, the defenders of your immune system.

☞ Helps regulate the immune response.

☞ May enhance the function of immune cells that protect against pathogens.

Research in the *Journal of Investigative Medicine* showed that vitamin D deficiency was associated with increased autoimmunity and susceptibility to infection. Sounds like a good reason to catch some rays (safely, of course).

SOURCES OF VITAMIN D

☞ Sunlight exposure

☞ Fatty fish

☞ Egg yolks

☞ Fortified foods

ZINC: THE IMMUNE SYSTEM'S LITTLE HELPER

Zinc is like the office assistant of your immune system; it helps keep everything running smoothly. Check out its resume.

☞ Helps develop and maintain immune cells.

☞ Necessary for wound healing.

☞ Supports the function of neutrophils and natural killer cells.

A meta-analysis published in the *American Journal of Clinical Nutrition* found that zinc supplementation reduced the duration and severity of common cold symptoms. Not too shabby for a little mineral.

SOURCES OF ZINC

- Oysters

- Beef

- Pumpkin seeds

- Lentils

- Yogurt

VITAMIN E: THE CELLULAR BODYGUARD

Vitamin E is like a bodyguard for your cells, protecting them from damage. Here's why it's important.

- Powerful antioxidant that helps protect immune cells.

- Enhances T cell function.

- May help protect against several infectious diseases.

A study in the *Journal of the American Medical Association* found that vitamin E supplementation improved certain clinically relevant measures of immune function in elderly individuals. It looks like this vitamin is fighting ageism in your immune system.

SOURCES OF VITAMIN E

- Nuts

- Seeds

- Avocados

- ⇗ Spinach

- ⇗ Butternut squash

PROTEIN: THE BUILDING BLOCKS OF IMMUNITY

Protein isn't just for muscle heads; it's crucial for your immune system too. Here's why.

- ⇗ Protein is necessary to produce antibodies.

- ⇗ It is essential for the proper functioning of immune cells.

- ⇗ Protein helps repair tissues, which is crucial during recovery from illness.

Research in the *British Journal of Nutrition* showed that even a modest deficiency in protein can impair immune function. So don't skimp on the protein, folks.

SOURCES OF PROTEIN

- ⇗ Lean meats

- ⇗ Fish

- ⇗ Eggs

- ⇗ Legumes

- ⇗ Nuts

- ⇗ Seeds

FOODS THAT SUPPORT THE IMMUNE SYSTEM
YOUR IMMUNITY GROCERY LIST

Now that we know the key nutrients, let's share some immune-boosting superfoods that should be on your shopping list.

GARLIC: THE STINKY IMMUNE BOOSTER

Garlic isn't just for warding off vampires; it's great for your immune system too. Here's why.

- ☞ Contains compounds that may help immune cells identify pathogens.

- ☞ Has antimicrobial and antiviral properties.

- ☞ May enhance the function of certain immune cells.

A study in *Advances in Therapy* found that participants taking garlic supplements had significantly fewer colds and recovered faster if they did get infected. Garlic breath might not be so bad after all.

MUSHROOMS: THE FUNGAL DEFENDERS

Mushrooms are like the undercover agents of the food world; they may not look like much, but they pack a powerful immune-boosting punch.

- ☞ Rich in beta-glucans, which can activate parts of your immune system.

- ☞ Good source of B vitamins and selenium, which support immune function.

- ☞ Some varieties, like shiitake, have been shown to improve immune markers.

Research in the *Journal of the American College of Nutrition* found that eating shiitake mushrooms daily improved immune function in healthy adults. Time to get fungi with it.

BERRIES: THE COLORFUL IMMUNE BOOSTERS

Berries aren't just delicious, they're like a multivitamin for your immune system.

- Rich in vitamin C and antioxidants.

- Contain anthocyanins, which have anti-inflammatory effects.

- May enhance the function of immune cells.

A study in *Nutrients* found that flavonoids from berries could enhance immune function and potentially reduce the incidence of upper respiratory tract infections. Berry, good news if you ask me.

FERMENTED FOODS: THE GUT-LOVING IMMUNE SUPPORTERS

Remember our chat about the gut-brain axis? Well, your gut plays a massive role in immunity too. Fermented foods can help in several ways.

- Support your gut health and, by extension, your immune system.

- They contain probiotics that support a healthy gut microbiome.

- May enhance the production of natural antibodies and can potentially reduce the risk of respiratory infections.

Research in the *British Journal of Nutrition* showed that consuming probiotic foods was associated with a lower incidence of upper respiratory tract infections. Yogurt for the win.

GREEN TEA: THE ANTIOXIDANT POWERHOUSE

Green tea isn't just for zen moments; it's a powerful immune supporter too.

- Rich in polyphenols, particularly EGCG, which have immune-boosting effects.

- May enhance the production of T cells.

- Has antimicrobial properties.

A study in the *Journal of the American College of Nutrition* found that green tea enhanced the proliferation of T cells and increased the production of antibodies. Time to put the kettle on.

DIETARY STRATEGIES
DURING COLD AND FLU SEASON
YOUR SEASONAL IMMUNITY GAME PLAN

When cold and flu season rolls around, it's time to kick your immune-boosting diet into high gear. Here are some strategies to help you weather the storm.

UP YOUR VITAMIN C INTAKE

While vitamin C might not prevent colds, research suggests it could reduce their duration and severity. A meta-analysis in the *Cochrane Database of Systematic Reviews* found that regular vitamin C supplementation reduced the duration of colds by 8% in adults and 14% in children.

> ☞ AIM TO INCLUDE VITAMIN C-RICH FOODS IN EVERY MEAL. Think oranges for breakfast, bell peppers in your lunch salad, and broccoli with dinner.

EMBRACE WARMING FOODS

Traditional wisdom often recommends warm foods during the cold season, and science backs this up. Warm foods like soups and broths can help maintain hydration and may help relieve congestion. A study in the journal *Chest* found that drinking hot chicken soup increased the movement of nasal mucus, potentially helping to relieve congestion. Chicken soup for more than just the soul.

> ☞ Incorporate warming soups and broths into your diet. Bonus points if they're packed with veggies and lean proteins.

GO FOR GARLIC AND ONIONS

These flavorful foods don't just make your dishes tastier. They're packed with immune-boosting compounds. A study in *Clinical Nutrition* found that aged garlic extract supplementation reduced the severity and duration of cold and flu symptoms. Talk about a pungent protector.

- ☞ Don't be shy with garlic and onions in your cooking. They're great additions to soups, stir-fries, and roasted vegetables.

SPICE IT UP!

Certain spices, like ginger and turmeric, have anti-inflammatory and antioxidant properties that may support immune function. Research in the *Journal of Ethnopharmacology* found that ginger effectively inhibited human respiratory syncytial virus, a common cause of respiratory infections. Spice up your life and your immune system.

- ☞ Try adding ginger to your tea or smoothies and incorporating turmeric into your cooking

  PRO TIP: Pair it with black pepper to enhance absorption).

STAY HYDRATED

Proper hydration is crucial for your health, including immune function. Water helps your body produce lymph, which carries white blood cells and other immune system cells. While there's no magic number for how much water you should drink, a good rule of thumb is to drink enough so that your urine is pale yellow.

- ☞ Keep a water bottle handy and sip throughout the day. Herbal teas can also contribute to your fluid intake.

PLEASE REMEMBER YOUR VITAMIN D

As daylight hours decrease in winter, many people become deficient in vitamin D, which can impact immune function. A systematic review in the *BMJ* found that vitamin D supplementation protected against acute respiratory tract infections, particularly in individuals who were very deficient.

- ☞ Consider having your vitamin D levels checked and discuss supplementation with your healthcare provider if needed. You can also include vitamin D-rich foods like fatty fish and egg yolks in your diet.

LIMIT ADDED SUGARS

High sugar intake can suppress immune function. A study in the *American Journal of Clinical Nutrition* found that consuming 100 g of sugar (equivalent to about two cans of soda) significantly reduced the ability of white blood cells to engulf bacteria.

> Be mindful of added sugars in your diet, particularly in processed foods and beverages. Opt for naturally sweet whole fruits instead of sugary snacks.

PRIORITIZE SLEEP

While not strictly a dietary strategy, good sleep is crucial for immune function and can impact your food choices. Lack of sleep can increase inflammation and reduce immune function. A study in *Sleep* found that individuals who slept less than 6 hours a night were four times more likely to catch a cold compared to those who slept more than 7 hours.

> AIM FOR 7–9 HOURS OF SLEEP PER NIGHT. Establish a relaxing bedtime routine and create a sleep-friendly environment.

BRINGING IT ALL TOGETHER
YOUR IMMUNE-BOOSTING ACTION PLAN

So, immunity warriors, are you ready to give your body's defense system the support it deserves? Here's a simple action plan to get you started.

EAT A RAINBOW
Aim to include a variety of colorful fruits and vegetables in your diet every day. This ensures you're getting a wide range of immune-boosting vitamins, minerals, and phytonutrients.

PRIORITIZE PROTEIN
Include a source of lean protein in each meal to support the production of immune cells and antibodies.

SPICE UP YOUR LIFE
Don't be afraid to use garlic, onions, ginger, and turmeric in your cooking. These flavorful additions pack a powerful immune-boosting punch.

STAY HYDRATED
Make water your beverage of choice and consider adding some immune-boosting herbal teas to your routine.

MIND YOUR GUT
Include fermented foods in your diet to support your gut microbiome and, by extension, your immune system.

SLEEP WELL
Prioritize getting enough quality sleep to give your immune system the rest it needs to function optimally.

MANAGE STRESS
While not directly related to diet, chronic stress can suppress immune function. Consider stress-management techniques like meditation or yoga.

Remember, boosting your immunity isn't about downing supplements or making drastic changes overnight. It's about consistently nourishing your body with immune-supporting foods and maintaining healthy lifestyle habits.

Your immune system is working hard for you 24/7, so show it some love with the fuel it needs to keep you healthy. Here's to a stronger, more resilient you.

CHAPTER 8

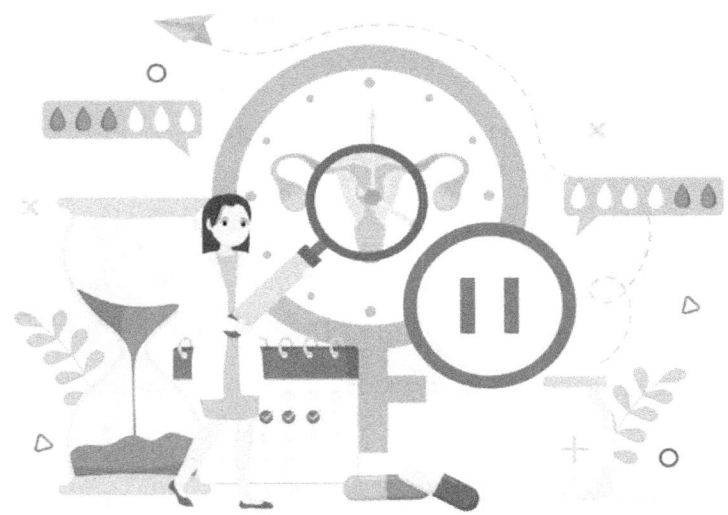

BALANCING HORMONES NATURALLY

EAT YOUR WAY TO HORMONAL HARMONY

Let's explore those chemical messengers that keep your body running like a well-oiled machine. Hormones are like the body's email system, sending important messages to your organs and tissues about everything from growth and metabolism to mood and reproduction. But what happens when this email system gets spammed or hacked? That's where hormone imbalances come in, and let me tell you, they can wreak havoc on your health faster than a computer virus.

The good news? Your diet can play a massive role in maintaining hormonal harmony. So, let's dive into how you can eat your way to better hormonal health.

ENDOCRINE DISRUPTORS IN FOOD
THE HORMONAL HACKERS

First things first, let's talk about the bad guys: endocrine disruptors. These are chemicals that can interfere with your body's hormonal system, potentially leading to developmental, reproductive, neurological, and immune problems. Yikes.

Here are some common endocrine disruptors that might be lurking in your food.

BISPHENOL A (BPA): THE CAN CULPRIT
BPA is like that annoying party crasher that shows up uninvited and causes chaos. It's found in:

☞ Canned foods (it's used in the lining of the cans),

☞ Plastic food containers,

☞ And plastic water bottles.

A study published in *Environmental Health Perspectives* found that people who ate one serving of canned soup daily for five days had a 1,000% increase in urinary BPA compared to those who ate fresh soup. That's one heck of a party crasher.

HOW TO AVOID IT
Opt for fresh or frozen foods instead of canned and choose glass or

stainless-steel containers over plastic.

PESTICIDES: THE PRODUCE POLLUTERS

Certain pesticides used in conventional farming can act as endocrine disruptors. These chemical gatecrashers can:

- ☞ Mimic or block hormones.

- ☞ Alter hormone production.

- ☞ Interfere with hormone signaling.

Research in the *International Journal of Andrology* found that some pesticides can affect male reproductive health by interfering with testosterone production. Not cool, pesticides. Not cool at all.

HOW TO AVOID THEM

Choose organic produce when possible, especially for the "Dirty Dozen" (fruits and vegetables known to have higher pesticide residues).

PHTHALATES: THE PLASTIC PERPETRATORS

Phthalates are like BPA's partners in crime. They're often found in:

- ☞ Plastic food packaging,

- ☞ And some personal care products.

A study in *Environment International* found that higher phthalate exposure was associated with increased insulin resistance and a higher body mass index in adolescents. These plastic perps are messing with our metabolism.

HOW TO AVOID THEM

- ☞ Limit use of plastic food containers (especially for hot foods).

- ☞ Choose personal care products labeled "phthalate-free".

ARTIFICIAL FOOD ADDITIVES: THE SYNTHETIC SABOTEURS

Some artificial food colors and preservatives have been linked to hormonal disruption. For example:

- Propyl gallate, used to prevent fats and oils from spoiling, may interfere with hormone function.

- Some artificial food colors have been linked to behavioral issues in children, which could be related to hormonal disruption.

A review in the *Journal of Clinical Endocrinology & Metabolism* highlighted how certain food additives could potentially interfere with hormonal processes.

HOW TO AVOID THEM

- Choose whole, unprocessed foods as much as possible, and read labels to avoid artificial additives.

DIETARY SUPPORT FOR HORMONAL HEALTH
FEEDING YOUR ENDOCRINE SYSTEM

Now that we've talked about what to avoid, let's focus on the good stuff—foods and nutrients that can support your hormonal health. We'll break this down by different areas of the endocrine system.

THYROID HEALTH: FUELING YOUR METABOLIC ENGINE

Your thyroid is like the thermostat of your body, regulating your metabolism. Here's how to keep it happy.

- IODINE is essential for thyroid hormone production. Sources include seaweed, fish, and iodized salt.

- SELENIUM helps activate thyroid hormones. Find it in Brazil: nuts, fish, and eggs.

☞ ZINC is crucial for thyroid hormone production. Good sources are oysters, beef, and pumpkin seeds.

A study in the *Journal of Clinical Endocrinology & Metabolism* found that mild iodine deficiency was associated with an increased risk of thyroid disorders So don't be shellfish; eat your seafood.

ADRENAL HEALTH: SUPPORTING YOUR STRESS RESPONSE

Your adrenal glands are like your body's emergency response team, producing stress hormones like cortisol. Here's how to support them:

☞ VITAMIN C is crucial for adrenal function. Find it in citrus fruits, bell peppers, and strawberries.

☞ B VITAMINS help your body cope with stress. Good sources are whole grains, lean meats, and leafy greens.

☞ MAGNESIUM helps regulate cortisol levels. Find it in nuts, seeds, and dark chocolate.

Research in *Nutrients* found that vitamin C supplementation reduced cortisol levels in marathon runners. So next time you're stressed, reach for an orange instead of the cookie jar.

REPRODUCTIVE HEALTH: BALANCING SEX HORMONES

Whether you're dealing with PMS, menopause, or just want to keep your reproductive system in top shape, here's what to eat:

☞ OMEGA-3 FATTY ACIDS help balance sex hormones. Find them in fatty fish, walnuts, and flaxseed.

☞ CRUCIFEROUS VEGETABLES contain compounds that help metabolize estrogen. Think broccoli, cauliflower, and Brussels sprouts.

☞ FIBER helps eliminate excess estrogen from the body. Good sources are whole grains, legumes, and fruits.

A study in the *American Journal of Clinical Nutrition* found that women who ate more omega-3 fatty acids had milder menopause symptoms. Fish for the win!

BLOOD SUGAR BALANCE: KEEPING INSULIN IN CHECK

Insulin is like the bouncer at the cellular club, deciding which nutrients get in. Here's how to keep it working smoothly:

- ☞ CINNAMON may help improve insulin sensitivity. Sprinkle it on your oatmeal or add to smoothies.

- ☞ CHROMIUM helps insulin do its job better. Find it in whole grains, broccoli, and grape juice.

- ☞ APPLE CIDER VINEGAR may help lower blood sugar levels. Try adding a splash to your salad dressing.

Research in the *Journal of Medicinal Food* found that cinnamon improved fasting blood glucose levels in people with type 2 diabetes. Spice up your life and your insulin sensitivity.

NUTRITION THROUGH DIFFERENT LIFE STAGES
HORMONAL SUPPORT FROM CRADLE TO GRAVE

Our hormonal needs change throughout our lives. Let's look at how to support hormonal health during different life stages:

PUBERTY: NAVIGATING THE HORMONAL ROLLER COASTER

Puberty is like your body's grand opening ceremony—numerous changes and a flood of new hormones. Here's how to support this transition:

HEALTHY FATS are essential for hormone production. Think avocados, nuts, and olive oil.

ZINC is important for reproductive development. Find it in oysters, beef, and pumpkin seeds.

IRON is crucial for girls starting menstruation. Good sources are lean meats, beans, and fortified cereals.

A study in the *Journal of Nutrition* found that higher intake of vegetable protein and fat during puberty was associated with later onset of menstruation, which is linked to a lower risk of breast cancer later in life. Plant power for the puberty win.

REPRODUCTIVE YEARS: SUPPORTING FERTILITY AND HORMONAL BALANCE

Whether you're trying to conceive or just want to keep your reproductive system humming, here's what to focus on:

FOLATE is crucial for fertility and fetal development. Find it in leafy greens, legumes, and fortified grains.

VITAMIN D is important for reproductive health. Get it from sunlight, fatty fish, and fortified foods.

ANTIOXIDANTS protect reproductive cells from damage. Colorful fruits and vegetables are your best bet.

Research in *Obstetrics & Gynecology* found that women who took a daily multivitamin had a 41% lower risk of ovulatory infertility. A little insurance policy for your fertility.

PREGNANCY: NOURISHING TWO (OR MORE)

Pregnancy is like hosting a very demanding guest for nine months. Here's how to keep everyone happy:

PROTEIN is essential for fetal growth. Aim for lean meats, fish, eggs, and plant-based sources like beans and lentils.

CALCIUM is crucial for bone development. Dairy products, leafy greens, and fortified foods are good sources.

OMEGA-3 FATTY ACIDS are essential for fetal brain development.

Fatty fish (in moderation), walnuts, and chia seeds are great options.

A study in the *American Journal of Clinical Nutrition* found that higher intake of omega-3s during pregnancy was associated with better problem-solving skills in children at age 6 months. Fish really is brain food.

MENOPAUSE: SMOOTHING THE TRANSITION

Menopause is like your body's retirement party for your reproductive system. Here's how to make it a good one:

PHYTOESTROGENS are plant compounds that may help balance hormones. Find them in soy products, flaxseeds, and sesame seeds.

CALCIUM AND VITAMIN D are crucial for bone health as estrogen levels decline. Dairy products, leafy greens, and fatty fish are good sources.

FIBER helps manage weight and blood sugar levels. Whole grains, fruits, and vegetables are your friends here.

Research in *Maturitas* found that a diet rich in whole grains, fruits, vegetables, and lean protein was associated with reduced menopause symptoms. Eat the rainbow to weather the menopause storm.

POST-MENOPAUSE: MAINTAINING HORMONAL HEALTH IN LATER YEARS

Just because the reproductive years are over doesn't mean hormonal health isn't relevant. Here's what to focus on:

PROTEIN helps maintain muscle mass. Aim for a mix of animal and plant-based proteins.

VITAMIN B12 is often poorly absorbed in older adults. Find it in lean meats, fish, and fortified foods.

ANTIOXIDANTS help fight age-related cellular damage. Berries, dark chocolate, and green tea are great sources.

A study in the *American Journal of Clinical Nutrition* found that higher protein intake was associated with a lower risk of frailty in older women. Protein power for the golden years.

BRINGING IT ALL TOGETHER
YOUR HORMONE-BALANCING GAME PLAN

Alright, hormone heroes, ready to take control of your endocrine email system? Here's a simple action plan to get you started.

DITCH THE DISRUPTORS
Minimize exposure to endocrine disruptors by choosing fresh, whole foods and avoiding plastic food containers when possible.

EAT THE RAINBOW
Aim for a variety of colorful fruits and vegetables to get a wide range of nutrients and antioxidants.

FOCUS ON HEALTHY FATS
Include sources of omega-3 fatty acids and other healthy fats in your diet to support hormone production.

PRIORITIZE PROTEIN
Make sure you're getting enough high-quality protein to support hormone synthesis and maintain muscle mass.

PLEASE NOTE FIBER
Include plenty of fiber-rich foods to help manage blood sugar and support digestive health.

SPICE IT UP
Incorporate hormone-supporting spices like cinnamon and turmeric into your meals.

STAY HYDRATED
Drink plenty of water to support all bodily functions, including hormone production and metabolism.

MIND YOUR MINERALS
Ensure you're getting enough iodine, selenium, and zinc to support thyroid function.

STRESS LESS

While not directly related to diet, managing stress through techniques like meditation or yoga can help balance cortisol levels.

TAILOR YOUR DIET TO YOUR LIFE STAGE

Remember that your nutritional needs change throughout life, so adjust your diet accordingly.

Remember, balancing your hormones isn't about quick fixes or magic pills. It's about consistently nourishing your body with hormone-supporting foods and maintaining healthy lifestyle habits.

Your endocrine system is working hard to keep your body in balance, so show it some love with the nutrients it needs to function optimally. Here's to hormonal harmony and a healthier, happier you.

A FINAL WORD ON HORMONES AND HEALTH

Before we wrap up this hormone-balancing bonanza, let's take a moment to appreciate just how amazing our endocrine system is. These chemical messengers orchestrate everything from our mood and energy levels to our growth and metabolism. They're the unsung heroes of our bodies, working tirelessly behind the scenes to keep us functioning.

But here's the thing, our modern lifestyle doesn't always make it easy for our hormones to do their job. From chronic stress to environmental toxins, our endocrine system faces many challenges. That's why it's so important to support it through our diet and lifestyle choices.

Remember, small changes can make a big difference when it comes to hormonal health. Maybe it's swapping out that plastic water bottle for a glass one or adding an extra serving of leafy greens to your day. Every little step counts.

And don't forget—while diet plays a crucial role in hormonal health, it's not the whole picture. Regular exercise, adequate sleep, stress management, and avoiding harmful substances like excessive alcohol and tobacco are all important pieces of the hormone-balancing puzzle.

Lastly, if you're experiencing symptoms of hormonal imbalance—things like irregular periods, unexplained weight changes, or mood swings—don't hesitate to talk to your healthcare provider. While diet can do wonders for hormonal health, sometimes additional support or medical intervention may be necessary.

So, here's to you, hormone heroes. May your endocrine email system run smoothly, your hormones stay in balance, and your body thank you for all the nourishing, hormone-supporting foods you feed it. Keep up the great work.

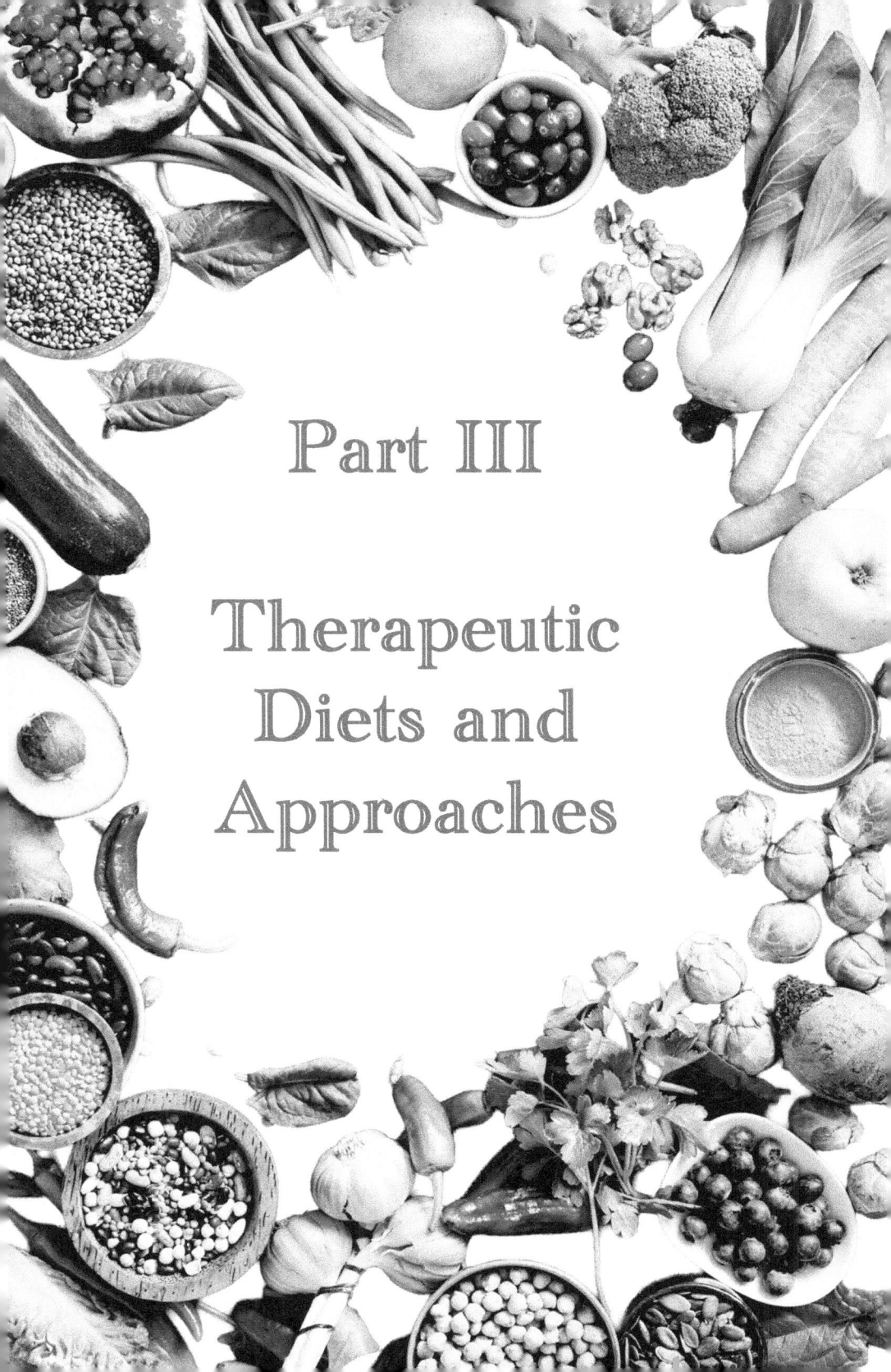

Part III

Therapeutic Diets and Approaches

CHAPTER 9

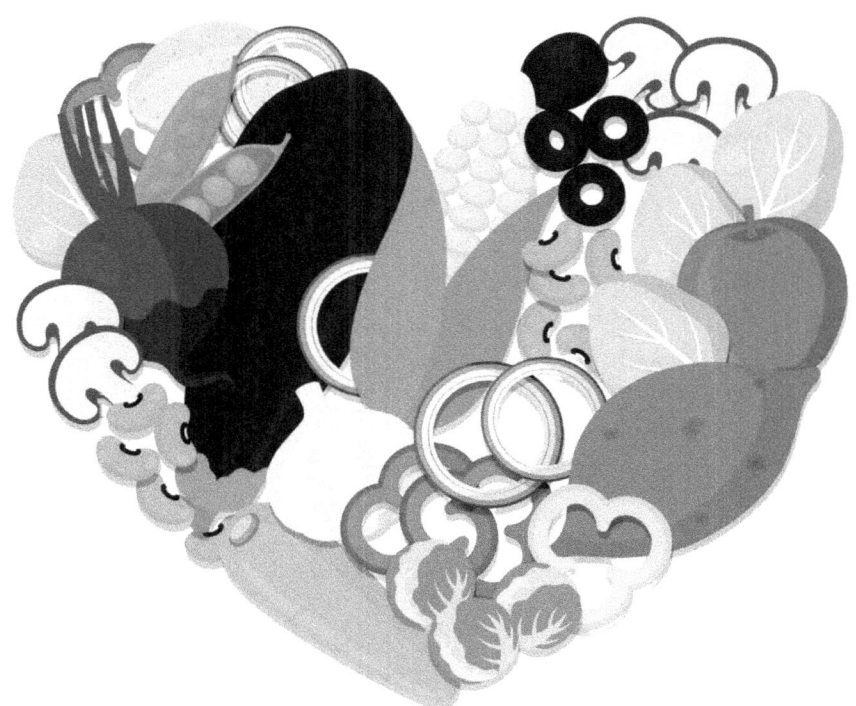

THE POWER OF PLANT-BASED EATING

UNLEASHING THE GREEN REVOLUTION

Veggie lovers and plant-curious pals. It's time to talk about one of the hottest trends in nutrition: plant-based eating. But don't worry, we're not here to turn you into a rabbit or shame you for enjoying a burger now and then. We're here to explore how adding more plants to your plate can supercharge your health, help the planet, and even make your taste buds do a happy dance. So, let's dig in and uncover the power of plants.

BENEFITS OF PLANT-BASED DIETS
WHY PLANTS PACK A PUNCH

First things first, let's talk about why plant-based diets are getting so much buzz. Spoiler alert: it's not just because they make for pretty Instagram posts (although that doesn't hurt).

HEART HEALTH: YOUR TICKER'S NEW BEST FRIEND
Plant-based diets are like a love letter to your heart. Here's why:

- Lower in saturated fat, which can help reduce cholesterol levels.

- Rich in fiber, which can help lower blood pressure and reduce heart disease risk.

- Packed with antioxidants that fight inflammation.

A landmark study published in the *Journal of the American Heart Association* found that following a plant-based diet was associated with a 16% lower risk of cardiovascular disease and a 32% lower risk of dying from cardiovascular disease. That's some serious plant power.

WEIGHT MANAGEMENT: SHEDDING POUNDS WITHOUT COUNTING CALORIES
If you've ever tried to lose weight by meticulously counting every calorie, you know it can be about as fun as watching paint dry. But are some cool things about plant-based diets:

- Lower in calories but higher in volume, helping you feel full on fewer calories.

⚘ Rich in fiber, which can increase satiety and reduce calorie intake.

⚘ Often leads to weight loss without the need for strict calorie counting.

A study in the *Journal of Geriatric Cardiology* found that people following a plant-based diet lost more weight than those following a non-vegetarian diet, even when they were allowed to eat until they were full. Talk about having your cake (made from zucchini, of course) and eating it too.

DIABETES MANAGEMENT: KEEPING YOUR BLOOD SUGAR IN CHECK

Plant-based diets can be a game-changer for managing or preventing type 2 diabetes. Here's why.

⚘ High in fiber, which slows down digestion and helps regulate blood sugar.

⚘ Often leads to improved insulin sensitivity.

⚘ Can help with weight management, a key factor in diabetes prevention and management.

Research published in *Diabetes Care* found that a low-fat vegan diet improved glycemic control and reduced the need for medications in people with type 2 diabetes. It's like giving your pancreas a high-five.

CANCER PREVENTION: FIGHTING THE BIG C WITH BROCCOLI (AND FRIENDS)

While no diet can guarantee cancer prevention, plant-based diets have shown some promising results.

⚘ Rich in antioxidants and phytochemicals that may help prevent cell damage.

⚘ High in fiber, which is associated with a lower risk of colorectal cancer.- Often leads to a healthier body weight, which is linked to lower cancer risk.

A comprehensive review in the *Journal of Geriatric Oncology* found that plant-based diets were associated with a lower risk of various types of cancer, including breast, colorectal, and prostate cancer. Vegetables: 1, Cancer: 0.

GUT HEALTH: FEEDING YOUR INTERNAL GARDEN

Remember our chat about the gut microbiome? Well, plant-based diets are like Miracle Gro for your good gut bacteria.

- High in prebiotic fiber, which feeds beneficial gut bacteria.

- Rich in diverse plant compounds that support a diverse microbiome.

- Often leads to increased production of short-chain fatty acids, which are beneficial for gut health.

A study in *Frontiers in Nutrition* found that plant-based diets can increase the diversity and health-promoting functions of gut microbiota. Happy gut, happy life.

ENVIRONMENTAL IMPACT: SAVING THE PLANET, ONE BITE AT A TIME

While this isn't directly related to your health, it's worth mentioning that plant-based diets can be a powerful tool in fighting climate change.

- Lower carbon footprint compared to diets high in animal products.

- Require less water and land use.

- Can help reduce deforestation and biodiversity loss.

A study in *Science* found that moving to a plant-based diet could reduce food-related emissions by up to 73%. Who knew your fork could be a weapon against climate change?

ENSURING NUTRITIONAL ADEQUACY
DODGING THE PITFALLS OF PLANT-BASED EATING

Now, before you go tossing all your steaks out the window, let's talk about how to make sure you're getting all the nutrients you need on a plant-based diet. Because, let's face it, living on nothing but potato chips and Oreos might technically be "plant-based," but it's not exactly a recipe for good health.

PROTEIN: THE BUILDING BLOCKS OF LIFE
Contrary to popular belief, you can absolutely get enough protein on a plant-based diet. Here's how.

- Legumes: beans, lentils, chickpeas (hello, hummus).

- Nuts and seeds: almonds, chia seeds, hemp seeds.

- Whole grains: quinoa, oats, wild rice.

- Soy products: tofu, tempeh, edamame.

PRO TIP: Combine different plant proteins throughout the day to ensure you're getting all essential amino acids.

A study in the *American Journal of Clinical Nutrition* found that dietary protein derived from plant sources is no less effective than animal protein in meeting human requirements. Take that, protein myths.

IRON: PUMPING IRON WITHOUT THE STEAK
Iron deficiency is a concern for many people, especially women. But fear not, plant-based iron sources are abundant.

- Leafy greens: spinach, kale, Swiss chard.

- Legumes: lentils, soybeans, kidney beans.

- Whole grains: quinoa, oatmeal, fortified cereals.

⚡ Dried fruits: raisins, apricots, prunes.

PRO TIP: Pair iron-rich foods with vitamin C sources (like citrus fruits or bell peppers) to enhance absorption.

Research in the *American Journal of Clinical Nutrition* showed that vegetarians are no more likely to have iron deficiency anemia than non-vegetarians. It's all about smart food choices.

VITAMIN B12: THE TRICKY ONE

B12 is primarily found in animal products, so it's the nutrient that plant-based eaters need to pay the most attention to. Here's how to get it.

⚡ Fortified plant milks and cereals.

⚡ Nutritional yeast.

⚡ B12 supplements (consult your healthcare provider).

A study in the *European Journal of Clinical Nutrition* found that vegans who don't take B12 supplements or eat fortified foods are at high risk of deficiency. Don't skimp on this one, folks.

CALCIUM: NOT JUST FOR DAIRY LOVERS

You don't need cow's milk to build strong bones. Here are some plant-based calcium sources.

⚡ Leafy greens: Kale, collard greens, Bok choy.

⚡ Fortified plant milks.

⚡ Tofu made with calcium sulfate.

⚡ Almonds and almond butter.

Research in the *American Journal of Clinical Nutrition* found that calcium absorption from some plant sources (like kale) can be even higher than from dairy. Green is the new white.

OMEGA-3 FATTY ACIDS: FISH AREN'T THE ONLY ONES IN THE SEA

While fish are often touted as the best source of omega-3s, plant-based eaters have options too.

- ☞ Flaxseeds and flaxseed oil.

- ☞ Chia seeds.

- ☞ Walnuts.

- ☞ Algae-based supplements.

A study in the *Journal of Nutrition* found that plant-based omega-3s can be effectively converted to the long-chain forms typically found in fish. It's all about giving your body the raw materials it requires.

TRANSITIONING TO A PLANT-BASED DIET
BABY STEPS TO SIGNIFICANT CHANGES

Alright, so you're convinced about the benefits of plant-based eating, and you know how to avoid nutritional pitfalls. But how do you actually make the switch without feeling overwhelmed? Here are some strategies to help you transition smoothly.

START WITH MEATLESS MONDAYS

Going plant-based doesn't have to be an all-or-nothing proposition. Start by designating one day a week as your plant-based day. It's like dipping your toe in the veggie pool before diving in.

A study in *Public Health Nutrition* found that even one day a week of plant-based eating can have significant health benefits. Every little bit counts.

CROWD OUT. DON'T CUT OUT

Instead of focusing on what you're eliminating, concentrate on adding more plant-based foods to your diet. As you add more veggies, fruits, whole grains, and legumes, you'll naturally have less room for animal products.

Research in the *International Journal of Obesity* found that increasing fruit and vegetable intake was associated with weight loss, even without specific instructions to reduce other foods. It's like magic, but with broccoli.

EXPLORE NEW FOODS AND CUISINES

Transitioning to a more plant-based diet is a great excuse to expand your culinary horizons. Try a new vegetable each week or explore cuisines that are naturally plant-heavy, like Indian or Mediterranean.

A study in the journal *Appetite* found that increasing variety in a plant-based diet was associated with greater adherence and enjoyment. Who says healthy eating must be boring?

REIMAGINE YOUR FAVORITE MEALS

You don't have to give up your favorite dishes. Get creative and find plant-based versions of your go-to meals. Love burgers? Try a black bean or lentil patty. Can't live without pizza? Load it up with veggies and use a cashew-based cheese.

Research in the *Journal of Nutrition Education and Behavior* found that providing familiar, "veganized" versions of popular dishes increased acceptance of plant-based meals. It's all about making the unfamiliar familiar.

STOCK YOUR PANTRY

Set yourself up for success by keeping your kitchen stocked with plant-based staples. Think canned beans, whole grains, nuts, seeds, and plenty of fruits and veggies.

A study in the *International Journal of Behavioral Nutrition and Physical Activity* found that having healthy foods readily available at home was associated with better dietary habits. Your environment shapes your choices.

BE KIND TO YOURSELF

Remember, transitioning to a more plant-based diet is a journey, not a destination. Don't beat yourself up if you're not perfect. Every plant-based meal is a win for your health and the planet.

Research in the *Journal of Health Psychology* found that self-compassion was associated with better adherence to health-promoting behaviors. Treat yourself like you would a good friend.

GET SUPPORT

Join a plant-based cooking class, find online communities, or get your friends and family involved. Having support can make the transition easier and more enjoyable.

A study in the *Annals of Behavioral Medicine* found that social support was a key factor in successful dietary changes. It takes a village to raise a plant-based eater.

BRINGING IT ALL TOGETHER
YOUR PLANT-BASED GAME PLAN

Alright, veggie voyagers, ready to embark on your plant-based adventure? Here's a simple action plan to get you started.

START SMALL
Choose one meal a day or one day a week to go plant-based.

FOCUS ON WHOLE FOODS
Prioritize fruits, vegetables, whole grains, legumes, nuts, and seeds.

EXPERIMENT IN THE KITCHEN
Try new recipes and plant-based versions of your favorite meals.

READ LABELS
Be aware of potential nutrient deficiencies and choose fortified foods or supplements if needed.

STAY HYDRATED
Drink plenty of water, especially as you increase your fiber intake.

LISTEN TO YOUR BODY
Pay attention to how different foods make you feel and adjust accordingly.

KEEP LEARNING
Stay informed about plant-based nutrition and cooking techniques.

Remember, the goal isn't perfection; it's progress. Whether you're going full vegan or just adding a few more plant-based meals to your week, you're taking steps towards better health for yourself and the planet. And that's something to celebrate.

A Final Thought
On Plant-Based Eating

As we wrap up our deep dive into the world of plant-based eating, let's take a moment to appreciate the incredible diversity and power of plants. From the humble bean to the mighty kale leaf, plants offer an astounding array of nutrients, flavors, and health benefits.

But beyond the nutritional aspects, embracing a more plant-based diet can be a profound shift in how we think about food, health, and our connection to the world around us. It's an opportunity to explore new cuisines, get creative in the kitchen, and even reduce our environmental footprint along the way.

Whether you're a longtime vegan, a curious omnivore, or somewhere in between, remember that there's no one-size-fits-all approach to nutrition. The key is finding a way of eating that nourishes your body, aligns with your values, and brings you joy.

So, here's to the power of plants—may your plate be colorful, your body be nourished, and your taste buds be delighted. Happy plant-based eating, everyone.

CHAPTER 10

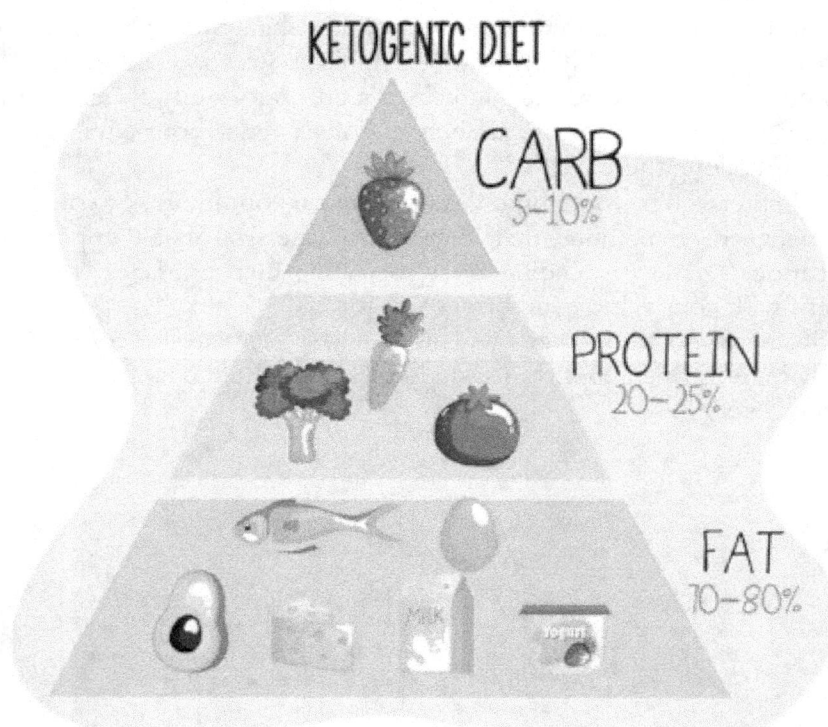

KETOGENIC DIETS

BENEFITS AND RISKS

Keto crusaders and curious carb-lovers. We will talk about one of the most buzzed-about diets of the past few years: the ketogenic diet. Now, before you roll your eyes and think, "Great, another fad diet," stick with me. We're going to dive deep into the science, explore some pretty cool potential benefits, and yes, talk about the risks too. Because let's face it, no diet is one-size-fits-all, and knowledge is power, baby.

THE SCIENCE BEHIND KETOSIS
YOUR BODY'S METABOLIC MAGIC TRICK

First things first, let's break down what happens in your body when you go keto. Prepare for a little bit of science, but I promise to keep it as fun as a Bill Nye episode.

THE CARB CRASH
BYE-BYE, GLUCOSE

The ketogenic diet is all about drastically reducing your carb intake—we're talking 20–50 grams per day, folks. That's like saying goodbye to your morning bagel and your lunchtime sandwich bread in one fell swoop. But why?

Well, normally, your body uses glucose (from carbs) as its primary fuel source. It's like your body is a car running on gasoline. But when you severely restrict carbs, you're cutting off the fuel supply. So, what does your clever body do? It switches to a different fuel source.

FAT TO THE RESCUE
HELLO, KETONES

When glucose is in short supply, your body starts breaking down fat for energy. But here's where it gets interesting: your liver takes some of that fat and turns it into ketones, which can be used for fuel by most of your body's cells, including your brain.

A study published in the journal *Nutrition & Metabolism* found that the brain can derive up to 70% of its energy from ketones during periods of glucose deprivation. It's like your body has a built-in backup generator.

KETOSIS
THE METABOLIC STATE OF FAT BURNING

When your body is primarily using ketones for fuel, you've entered a state called ketosis. It's like your metabolism has shifted gears, becoming a fat-burning machine.

Research in the journal *Obesity Reviews* showed that ketosis can increase energy expenditure and fat oxidation. In other words, you're burning more calories and more fat just by being in this state. Talk about working smarter, not harder.

INSULIN
THE HORMONE THAT TAKES A BACK SEAT

Here's another cool thing about ketosis: it leads to lower insulin levels. Insulin is the hormone that helps shuttle glucose into your cells, but it also promotes fat storage. When insulin levels drop, it becomes easier for your body to access and burn stored fat.

A study in the journal *Diabetes & Metabolic Syndrome* found that a ketogenic diet significantly reduced insulin levels in overweight individuals with type 2 diabetes. It's like giving your pancreas a well-deserved vacation.

POTENTIAL THERAPEUTIC APPLICATIONS
KETO'S SUPERPOWERS

Now that we understand the basics of how ketosis works, let's explore some potential health benefits. Spoiler alert: it's not just about weight loss.

WEIGHT MANAGEMENT: SHEDDING POUNDS WITHOUT HUNGER PANGS

One of the most well-known benefits of the ketogenic diet is its effectiveness for weight loss. But it's not just about cutting calories. Here's why keto can be a weight loss powerhouse.

> ☟ INCREASED SATIETY: Fat and protein are more filling than carbs, helping you feel full on fewer calories.

⚕ REDUCED CRAVINGS: Stable blood sugar levels can help reduce those pesky sugar cravings.

⚕ PRESERVED MUSCLE MASS: The high protein intake helps maintain muscle while losing fat.

A meta-analysis published in the *British Journal of Nutrition* found that individuals following a ketogenic diet achieved greater long-term weight loss compared to those on low-fat diets. It's like your body becomes a fat-burning furnace.

EPILEPSY MANAGEMENT: THE ORIGINAL KETO SUPERPOWER

Did you know that the ketogenic diet was originally developed in the 1920s as a treatment for epilepsy? It's true. And it's still used today, especially for children with drug-resistant epilepsy.

A review in the journal *Neurology* found that about half of children with epilepsy who follow a ketogenic diet experience a 50% or greater reduction in seizures. For some, it can be life-changing.

TYPE 2 DIABETES: TAMING THE BLOOD SUGAR ROLLER COASTER

The ketogenic diet's ability to lower blood sugar and insulin levels makes it a potential game-changer for managing type 2 diabetes. Improved insulin sensitivity: Your cells become more responsive to insulin.

⚕ REDUCED MEDICATION NEEDS: Some people can reduce or even eliminate diabetes medications.

⚕ BETTER BLOOD SUGAR CONTROL: Fewer carbs mean fewer blood sugar spikes.

A study in the journal *Nutrition & Metabolism* found that after 24 weeks on a ketogenic diet, 95% of participants with type 2 diabetes reduced or eliminated their glucose-lowering medications. Now that's what I call a diabetes diet revolution.

NEUROLOGICAL DISORDERS: FEEDING YOUR BRAIN'S PREFERRED FUEL

Emerging research suggests that the ketogenic diet might have neuroprotective effects, potentially benefiting conditions like Alzheimer's, Parkinson's, and traumatic brain injury. Improved mitochondrial function: Ketones provide efficient energy for brain cells.

⚮ Reduced oxidative stress: Ketones have antioxidant properties.

⚮ Enhanced brain-derived neurotrophic factor (BDNF): This protein supports the survival of existing neurons and encourages the growth of new ones.

A study in the journal *Neurobiology of Aging* found that a ketogenic diet improved cognitive performance in older adults at risk for Alzheimer's disease. It's like giving your brain a tune-up.

CANCER: A POTENTIAL ALLY IN TREATMENT

While more research is needed, some studies suggest that the ketogenic diet might be beneficial as an adjunct to cancer treatment. Starving cancer cells: Many cancer cells rely heavily on glucose for fuel and can't effectively use ketones.

⚮ Reducing inflammation: Chronic inflammation is linked to cancer development and progression.

⚮ Enhancing the effects of some cancer therapies: Some research suggests keto might make certain cancer cells more vulnerable to treatment.

A pilot study published in *Nutrition & Metabolism* found that combining a ketogenic diet with standard treatments for patients with advanced metastatic tumors resulted in stable disease or partial remission in 5 out of 16 patients. While not a cure, it's an exciting area of research.

POLYCYSTIC OVARY SYNDROME (PCOS): BALANCING HORMONES NATURALLY

PCOS, a hormonal disorder common among women of reproductive age, might also benefit from a ketogenic approach. Improved insulin sensitivity: PCOS is often associated with insulin resistance.

⌖ Weight loss: Many women with PCOS struggle with weight management.

⌖ Reduced testosterone levels: High testosterone is a hallmark of PCOS.

A small study in the *Journal of Translational Medicine* found that women with PCOS who followed a ketogenic diet for 24 weeks saw significant improvements in weight, hormone levels, and fasting insulin. It's like giving your ovaries a helping hand.

LONG-TERM
CONSIDERATIONS AND PRECAUTIONS
THE KETO CATCH

Now, before you go tossing all your bread in the trash, let's talk about some potential downsides and precautions of long-term keto eating. Because, as with any diet, it's not all sunshine and bacon roses.

THE KETO FLU: THE INITIATION PROCESS

When you first start a ketogenic diet, you might experience what's known as the "keto flu." It's not actually the flu, but a collection of symptoms that can occur as your body adjusts to using ketones for fuel.

⌖ Fatigue.

⌖ Headaches.

⌖ Nausea.

⌖ Dizziness.

⌖ Irritability.

PRO TIP: Stay hydrated and make sure you're getting enough electrolytes during this transition period.

The good news? These symptoms usually subside after a few days to a couple of weeks. Think of it as your body's way of hazing you into the keto club.

NUTRIENT DEFICIENCIES: MIND THE GAPS

The restrictive nature of the ketogenic diet can make it challenging to get all the nutrients your body needs.

   ☞ FIBER: Many high-fiber foods are also high in carbs.

   ☞ CERTAIN VITAMINS AND MINERALS: Especially those found in fruits and whole grains.

PRO TIP: Consider taking a high-quality multivitamin and focusing on nutrient-dense, low-carb foods like leafy greens, avocados, and nuts.

A study in the journal *Nutrients* found that long-term ketogenic dieters were at risk for deficiencies in vitamins A, C, K, and folate, as well as calcium, magnesium, and potassium.

KIDNEY STONES: A ROCKY SIDE EFFECT

Some long-term keto dieters may be at increased risk for kidney stones. High protein intake can increase uric acid production. Inadequate fluid intake can concentrate urine.

Research in the journal *Pediatrics* found that about one in twenty children on long-term ketogenic diets for epilepsy developed kidney stones.

PRO TIP: Stay well-hydrated and consider discussing potassium citrate supplementation with your healthcare provider if you're at risk.

LIPID PROFILE CHANGES: THE CHOLESTEROL CONUNDRUM

The high fat content of the ketogenic diet can lead to changes in blood lipid levels. Increased LDL cholesterol is often called "bad" cholesterol.

- ⚐ INCREASED HDL CHOLESTEROL: Often called "good" cholesterol.

- ⚐ DECREASED TRIGLYCERIDES: A type of fat in your blood.

  PRO TIP: Regular lipid panel testing is important if you're following a long-term ketogenic diet, especially if you have a history of heart disease.

A meta-analysis in the *British Journal of Nutrition* found that while ketogenic diets typically increase HDL and decrease triglycerides, the effect on LDL can vary widely between individuals.

GUT MICROBIOME CHANGES: FEEDING YOUR INTERNAL ECOSYSTEM

The drastic reduction in carbs, including fiber, can lead to changes in your gut microbiome.

- ☞ Decreased diversity of gut bacteria.

- ☞ Potential increase in inflammation-promoting bacteria.

  PRO TIP: Focus on including low-carb sources of prebiotic fiber like asparagus, garlic, and onions, and consider a probiotic supplement.

A study in the journal *Applied and Environmental Microbiology* found that a ketogenic diet led to significant changes in the gut microbiome of mice, including a decrease in beneficial Bifidobacteria.

COMPLIANCE CHALLENGES: THE SOCIAL AND PRACTICAL HURDLES

Let's face it, following a strict ketogenic diet in our carb-centric world can be challenging.

☞ SOCIAL SITUATIONS: Try explaining to Grandma why you can't eat her famous mashed potatoes at Thanksgiving.

☞ MEAL PLANNING AND PREPARATION: It takes effort to constantly plan and prepare keto-friendly meals.

☞ POTENTIAL FOR DISORDERED EATING: The restrictive nature of the diet can trigger or exacerbate disordered eating patterns in susceptible individuals.

PRO TIP: Consider a cyclical or targeted ketogenic approach, where you incorporate higher-carb days or meals around workouts, to improve long-term sustainability.

A study in the journal *Nutrients* found that adherence to a ketogenic diet tends to decrease over time, with many people finding it difficult to maintain long-term.

MEDICAL CONSIDERATIONS: WHEN KETO MIGHT NOT BE YOUR FRIEND

While the ketogenic diet can be beneficial for many, it's not suitable for everyone. It may be contraindicated or require close medical supervision for people with:

☞ Pancreatic disease.

☞ Liver conditions.

☞ Gallbladder disease.

☞ History of eating disorders.

☞ Certain rare metabolic disorders.

Always consult a healthcare provider before starting a ketogenic diet, especially if you have any pre-existing health conditions or are taking medications.

Bringing It All Together
Your Keto Consideration Checklist

Alright, keto curious folks, let's recap and put together a checklist to help you decide if the ketogenic diet might be right for you.

- ASSESS YOUR GOALS: Is keto aligned with your health and wellness objectives?

- CONSULT A PROFESSIONAL: Talk to your healthcare provider, especially if you have any pre-existing conditions.

- PLAN FOR THE TRANSITION: Be prepared for potential "keto flu" symptoms and how to manage them.

- FOCUS ON NUTRIENT DENSITY: Choose high-quality, nutrient-rich foods within the keto framework.

- MONITOR YOUR HEALTH: Regular check-ups and blood tests are important for long-term keto dieters.

- CONSIDER SUPPLEMENTATION: A multivitamin, electrolytes, and probiotics may be beneficial.

- PLAN FOR SOCIAL SITUATIONS: Think about how you'll handle dining out and social events.

- LISTEN TO YOUR BODY: Pay attention to how you feel and be willing to adjust your approach if needed.

- THINK LONG-TERM: Consider whether a strict ketogenic diet is sustainable for you or if a modified approach might be more realistic.

- STAY INFORMED: Keep up with the latest research on ketogenic diets and their health effects.

A Final Thought
on Ketogenic Diets

As we wrap up our journey through the land of ketones and low-carb living, it's important to remember that the ketogenic diet, like any dietary approach, is a tool. For some, it can be a powerful one, offering benefits ranging from weight loss to improved neurological health. Others may not be the right fit.

The key is to approach any dietary change with an open mind, a willingness to listen to your body, and a commitment to making informed, health-focused decisions. Whether you decide to go full keto, try a modified version, or stick with a different eating style altogether, the most important thing is finding an approach that nourishes your body, supports your health goals, and fits into your lifestyle.

Remember, your dietary choices are just one part of the bigger picture of health. Regular physical activity, stress management, good sleep habits, and joyful living all play crucial roles in your wellbeing.

So, here's to making informed choices, listening to our bodies, and finding the dietary approach that helps us feel our best. May your journey be filled with health, happiness, and maybe just a little bit of butter coffee (if that's your thing).

CHAPTER 11

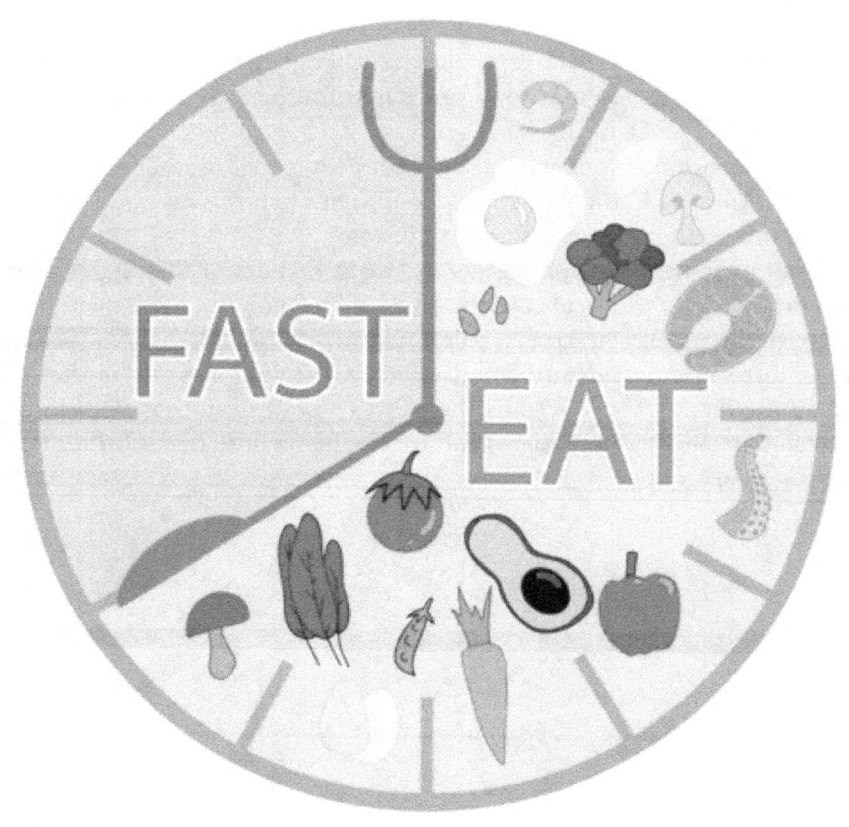

INTERMITTENT FASTING AS A HEALING TOOL

Timing is everything. Food-timing fanatics and curious meal-skippers. It's time to talk about one of the hottest trends in the nutrition world: intermittent fasting. Now, before you start panicking about going hungry, let me assure you—this isn't about starving yourself. It's about strategically timing when you eat. So, grab a glass of water (because that's always allowed.) and let's dive into the world of intermittent fasting.

DIFFERENT FASTING PROTOCOLS
PICK YOUR FASTING FLAVOR

First things first, let's break down the different types of intermittent fasting. Because, let's face it, one size doesn't fit all when it comes to not eating.

THE 16/8 METHOD: THE "SKIPPING BREAKFAST" APPROACH

This is the most popular form of intermittent fasting. Here's how it works.

- Fast for 16 hours a day.

- Eat all your meals within an 8-hour window. For example, you might eat between 12 pm and 8 pm, then fast from 8 pm to 12 pm the next day.

It's like giving your digestive system the night shifts off.

THE 5:2 DIET: THE "PART-TIME" FAST

This approach involves eating normally five days a week and significantly reducing calories on the other two days.

- Eat normally for five days.

- Consume only 500-600 calories on two non-consecutive days.

It's like putting your metabolism on a part-time job.

EAT-STOP-EAT: THE "24-HOUR CHALLENGE"
This method involves a full 24-hour fast, once or twice a week.

- Fast for 24 hours, from dinner one day to dinner the next day.

- Eat normally on non-fasting days.

Think of it as giving your digestive system a day off work.

THE WARRIORS DIET: THE "UNDEREATING AND OVEREATING" CYCLE
This protocol involves eating very little during the day and having one large meal at night.

- Eat small amounts of raw fruits and vegetables during the day.

- Have one large meal in the evening.

It's like being a dietary night owl.

ALTERNATE-DAY FASTING: THE "EVERY OTHER DAY" APPROACH
This method alternates between "fasting" days and regular eating days.

- Eat very little (about 500 calories) one day.

- Eat normally the next day.

It's like playing dietary hopscotch.

POTENTIAL HEALTH BENEFITS
FASTING'S SUPERPOWERS

Now that we know the different flavors of fasting, let's talk about why people are getting so excited about it. Spoiler alert: it's not just about weight loss.

WEIGHT LOSS AND FAT BURNING: SHEDDING POUNDS WITHOUT COUNTING CALORIES

One of the most popular reasons people try intermittent fasting is for weight loss. Here's why it can be effective.

- ⚐ REDUCED CALORIE INTAKE: You're simply eating less often.

- ⚐ INCREASED FAT BURNING: Fasting can boost your metabolic rate.

A study published in the journal *Obesity* found that alternate-day fasting was effective for weight loss and cardiovascular protection in both normal-weight and overweight adults. Fasting for the win.

INSULIN SENSITIVITY: TAMING THE BLOOD SUGAR ROLLER COASTER

Intermittent fasting can have powerful effects on insulin levels and insulin sensitivity.

- ⚐ LOWER INSULIN LEVELS: Fasting periods allow insulin levels to drop.

- ⚐ IMPROVED INSULIN SENSITIVITY: Your cells become more responsive to insulin.

Research in the journal *Cell Metabolism* showed that intermittent fasting could improve insulin sensitivity even without weight loss. It's like giving your pancreas a tune-up.

CELLULAR REPAIR: SPRING CLEANING FOR YOUR CELLS

During fasting periods, your cells initiate cellular repair processes, including autophagy.

- ⚐ AUTOPHAGY: Your cells break down and recycle old, damaged proteins.

↪ INCREASED GROWTH HORMONE: This can aid in fat loss and muscle gain.

A study in the journal *Autophagy* found that fasting could induce profound neuronal autophagy, potentially protecting against neurodegenerative diseases. It's like giving your brain cells a spa day.

HEART HEALTH: KEEPING YOUR TICKER IN TOP SHAPE
Intermittent fasting may improve various risk factors for heart disease.

↪ Lower blood pressure.

↪ Reduced "bad" LDL cholesterol and triglycerides.

↪ Decreased inflammation markers.

Research in the *American Journal of Clinical Nutrition* found that alternate-day fasting improved cardiovascular risk markers in overweight adults. Your heart might just thank you for skipping a meal or two.

BRAIN HEALTH: FEEDING YOUR MIND BY NOT FEEDING
Intermittent fasting might be good for your brain too.

↪ Increased production of brain-derived neurotrophic factor (BDNF).

↪ Potential protection against neurodegenerative diseases.

↪ Possible improvement in mood and focus.

A review in the journal *Ageing Research Reviews* suggested that intermittent fasting could enhance cognitive performance and protect against age-related cognitive decline. Who knew not eating could be food for thought?

LONGEVITY: LIVING LONGER BY EATING LESS OFTEN
While we can't say for sure that intermittent fasting will help you live longer (we'd need a long study for that),. Animal research is promising.

↬ Extended lifespan in various species.

↬ Improved markers of aging.

A study in *Cell Metabolism* found that mice subjected to intermittent fasting lived longer and had lower rates of cancer compared to mice that ate whenever they wanted. There's something to that old saying, "Leave the table a little hungry".

THE FASTING STUDY SPOTLIGHT
FASTING FOR METABOLIC HEALTH

Let's zoom in on a fascinating study that really showcases the potential of intermittent fasting. Published in the journal *Cell Metabolism* in 2019, this study looked at the effects of early time-restricted feeding (eTRF), a form of intermittent fasting where all meals are fit into an early 6-hour period of the day (e.g., 8 am to 2 pm).

The researchers found that eTRF improved insulin sensitivity, blood pressure, oxidative stress, and appetite. Participants also had significantly lower levels of the hunger hormone ghrelin in the morning and increased feelings of fullness in the evening.

What's really cool about this study is that these benefits were seen even when participants ate the same number of calories as the control group. It wasn't about eating less, but about timing those meals earlier in the day.

The lead author, Dr. Courtney Peterson, noted, "We found that eating early in the day to be more in sync with circadian rhythms appears to reduce body fat and improve health."

So, it seems like when you eat might be just as important as what you eat. It's like your body has an internal clock, and syncing your meals with it could be a game-changer for your health.

WHO SHOULD (AND SHOULDN'T) TRY INTERMITTENT FASTING: IS IT RIGHT FOR YOU?

Alright, before you start setting your eating times, let's talk about who might benefit from intermittent fasting and who should probably stick to regular mealtimes.

WHO MIGHT BENEFIT

- Healthy adults looking to lose weight or improve metabolic health.

- People at risk for type 2 diabetes or cardiovascular disease.

- Those looking to simplify their eating habits and reduce meal planning stress.

- Individuals interested in potential cognitive and anti-aging benefits.

WHO SHOULD BE CAUTIOUS OR AVOID INTERMITTENT FASTING?

- Pregnant or breastfeeding women.

- Children and teenagers.

- People with a history of eating disorders.

- Individuals with diabetes (especially type 1) should only fast under close medical supervision.

- Those on certain medications that need to be taken with food.

- People who are underweight or have a history of malnutrition.

Remember, even if you fall into the "might benefit" category, it's always a good idea to chat with your healthcare provider before starting any new eating pattern, especially one as different as intermittent fasting.

POTENTIAL ISSUES AND SIDE EFFECTS
THE FASTING FINE PRINT

Now, let's talk about some potential downsides of intermittent fasting.

Because, let's face it, no eating pattern is perfect for everyone.

HUNGER AND IRRITABILITY: THE HANGRY IS REAL

Especially when you're first starting out, you might experience some of these symptoms.

- Increased hunger.

- Irritability or "hanger".

- Difficulty concentrating.

These symptoms usually improve as your body adapts to the new eating pattern. Think of it as your stomach throwing a tantrum because it's not getting its usual snacks.

OVEREATING DURING EATING WINDOWS: THE FEAST OR FAMINE EFFECT

Some people might find themselves overeating during their eating windows, which can negate the benefits of fasting.

- Consuming excess calories.

- Making poor food choices due to extreme hunger.

It's important to still focus on nutrient-dense, balanced meals during your eating periods. Quality still matters.

NUTRIENT DEFICIENCIES: MIND THE GAPS

If you're not careful, restricting your eating window can make it challenging to get all the nutrients your body needs.

- Reduced overall food intake.

- Potential for limited dietary variety.

A varied, nutrient-dense diet is crucial, even when practicing intermittent fasting. It's about timing your nutrients, not eliminating them.

SOCIAL CHALLENGES: THE "SORRY, I'M FASTING" SCENARIO

Intermittent fasting can make social situations around food a bit tricky.

- Missing out on shared meals.

- Explaining your eating pattern to friends and family.

Flexibility is key—it's okay to adjust your fasting schedule for special occasions.

IMPACT ON EXERCISE: FUELING YOUR WORKOUTS

Some people might find it challenging to exercise during fasted periods. Reduced energy levels.

- Potential for decreased performance

Timing your workouts with your eating windows might help, or you might need to adjust your fasting schedule to accommodate your exercise routine.

HORMONAL CHANGES: LADIES, LISTEN UP

- Some women may experience changes in their menstrual cycles when starting intermittent fasting—irregular periods.

- Some women may experience fertility changes.

If you notice any significant changes, it's important to check in with your healthcare provider.

BRINGING IT ALL TOGETHER
YOUR INTERMITTENT FASTING ACTION PLAN

Alright, fasting curious folks, ready to give it a try? Here's a simple action plan to get you started.

- ☞ CHOOSE YOUR PROTOCOL: Pick the fasting method that best fits your lifestyle and goals.

- ☞ START SLOW: Begin with a less intense form of fasting and gradually increase as your body adapts.

- ☞ STAY HYDRATED: Drink plenty of water, especially during fasting periods.

- ☞ FOCUS ON NUTRIENT-DENSE FOODS: Make sure your meals during eating windows are balanced and nutritious.

- ☞ LISTEN TO YOUR BODY: Pay attention to how you feel and be willing to adjust your approach if needed.

- ☞ BE FLEXIBLE: It's okay to modify your fasting schedule for special occasions or when your body requires it.

- ☞ TRACK YOUR PROGRESS: Keep a journal of how you feel, any changes in weight or health markers, and your full experience.

- ☞ CONSULT A PROFESSIONAL: Check in with your healthcare provider, especially if you have any pre-existing health conditions.

Remember, intermittent fasting is a tool, not a magic bullet. It can be a powerful approach for some, but it's not right for everyone. The key is to find an eating pattern that supports your health goals, fits your lifestyle, and makes you feel good.

A FINAL THOUGHT
ON INTERMITTENT FASTING

As we wrap up our exploration of intermittent fasting, it's worth noting that this approach to eating is as much about when you eat as it is about what you eat. It's a different way of thinking about nutrition that challenges the conventional wisdom of "three square meals a day."

For some, intermittent fasting can be a game-changer, offering benefits ranging from weight loss to improved metabolic health. Others might not be the right fit. And that's okay. The most important thing is finding an approach to eating that nourishes your body, supports your health goals, and fits into your lifestyle.

Remember, your dietary choices are just one part of the bigger picture of health. Regular physical activity, stress management, good sleep habits, and joyful living all play crucial roles in your wellbeing.

So, here's to exploring new approaches to eating, listening to our bodies, and finding the nutritional strategy that helps us feel our best. May your journey with food, whether it involves fasting or not, be one of discovery, health, and happiness.

CHAPTER 12

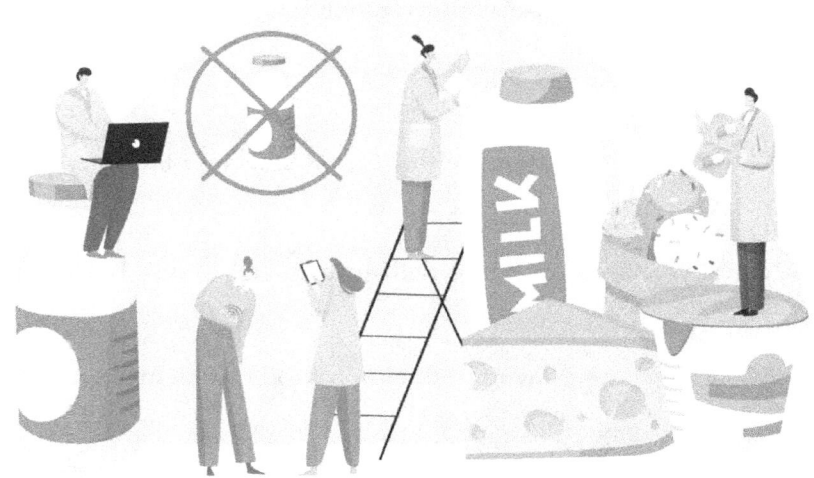

ELIMINATION DIETS AND FOOD SENSITIVITIES

DECODING YOUR BODY'S FOOD CLUES

Put on our detective hats and dive into the mysterious world of food allergies, intolerances, and sensitivities. Ever wonder why certain foods make you feel like you've been hit by a truck? Or why your best friend can chow down on peanuts while you break out in hives at the mere thought of them? Well, buckle up, because we're about to embark on a journey through the land of elimination diets and food sensitivities.

COMMON FOOD ALLERGIES AND INTOLERANCES
THE USUAL SUSPECTS

First things first, let's break down the difference between food allergies and intolerances.

FOOD ALLERGY
An immune system response that can be severe or life-threatening.

FOOD INTOLERANCE
A digestive system response that's usually less severe but can still be uncomfortable.

Now, let's meet our lineup of common food troublemakers.

THE "BIG EIGHT" FOOD ALLERGENS
These eight foods account for about 90% of all food allergies.

MILK: The most common food allergy in infants and young children.

> ☞ SYMPTOMS: Hives, wheezing, vomiting, digestive issues.

> ☞ HIDDEN SOURCES: Casein, whey, lactose.

EGGS: Another common allergen, especially in children.

> ☞ SYMPTOMS: Skin reactions, digestive issues, anaphylaxis in severe cases.

☞ HIDDEN SOURCES: Albumin, globulin, ovalbumin.

PEANUTS: One of the most common causes of severe allergic reactions.

☞ SYMPTOMS: Hives, swelling, difficulty breathing, anaphylaxis.

☞ HIDDEN SOURCES: Peanut oil, ground nuts, artificial nuts.

TREE NUTS: Includes almonds, cashews, walnuts, and more.

☞ SYMPTOMS: Hives, swelling, difficulty breathing, anaphylaxis.

☞ HIDDEN SOURCES: Nut butters, nut oils, marzipan.

FISH: Can cause severe allergic reactions.

☞ SYMPTOMS: Hives, wheezing, vomiting, dizziness.

☞ HIDDEN SOURCES: Fish sauce, Caesar dressing, Worcestershire sauce.

SHELLFISH: Includes shrimp, crab, lobster, and more.

☞ SYMPTOMS: Hives, wheezing, vomiting, anaphylaxis.

☞ HIDDEN SOURCES: Fish stock, seafood flavoring.

SOY: Common in many processed foods.

☞ SYMPTOMS: Tingling in the mouth, hives, itching, eczema.

☞ HIDDEN SOURCES: Tofu, tempeh, edamame, and some vegetable oils.

WHEAT: Can be confused with celiac disease or gluten sensitivity.

☞ SYMPTOMS: Hives, digestive issues, anaphylaxis in severe cases.

☞ HIDDEN SOURCES: Flour, breadcrumbs, some sauces, and gravies.

FUN FACT: A study published in the *Journal of Allergy and Clinical Immunology* found that about 32 million Americans have food allergies, including 5.6 million children. That's a lot of EpiPens!

OTHER COMMON FOOD INTOLERANCES

While not as severe as allergies, these can still cause significant discomfort.

LACTOSE INTOLERANCE: Difficulty digesting the sugar in milk.

☞ SYMPTOMS: Bloating, gas, diarrhea.

☞ HIDDEN SOURCES: Milk, cheese, ice cream, some medications.

GLUTEN SENSITIVITY: Different from celiac disease but can cause similar symptoms.

☞ SYMPTOMS: Bloating, abdominal pain, fatigue, headaches.

☞ HIDDEN SOURCES: Wheat, barley, rye, and some oats.

FODMAPS: fermentable oligosaccharides, disaccharides, monosaccharides, and polyols.

☞ SYMPTOMS: Bloating, gas, abdominal pain.

☞ COMMON CULPRITS: Certain fruits, vegetables, dairy products, and sweeteners.

HISTAMINE INTOLERANCE: Difficulty breaking down histamine in foods.

- SYMPTOMS: Headaches, flushing, itching, digestive issues.

- HIGH-HISTAMINE FOODS: Aged cheeses, fermented foods, cured meats, certain fish.

SULFITE SENSITIVITY: Reaction to sulfites used as preservatives.

- SYMPTOMS: Wheezing, coughing, chest tightness.

- COMMON SOURCES: Wine, dried fruits, some processed foods.

A study in the journal *Nutrients* found that up to 20% of the population may suffer from food intolerances, although many go undiagnosed. It's like having a secret food nemesis.

HOW TO CONDUCT AN ELIMINATION DIET
YOUR FOOD DETECTIVE TOOLKIT

Alright, now that we know the usual suspects, let's talk about how to figure out if any of these troublemakers are causing your symptoms. Enter the elimination diet—your personal food investigation tool.

STEP 1: PREPARE FOR YOUR FOOD DETECTIVE WORK
Before you start eliminating foods, do some prep work.

- Keep a food and symptom diary for a week or two.

- Make a list of suspect foods based on common allergens and your symptoms.

- Plan your meals for the elimination phase.

- Stock up on "safe" foods.

☞ Inform your family and friends about your diet plan.

PRO TIP: A study in the journal *Gastroenterology Nursing* found that keeping a detailed food and symptom diary can significantly improve the accuracy of food intolerance diagnosis. It's like being your CSI: Food Unit.

STEP 2: THE ELIMINATION PHASE
This is where the real detective work begins.

☞ Remove all suspect foods from your diet for 2-4 weeks.

☞ Be vigilant about reading labels and avoiding hidden sources.

☞ Continue to keep your food and symptom diary.

☞ Pay attention to how you feel—energy levels, digestion, skin, etc.

Remember, you're not just eliminating individual foods, but entire food groups that might contain your triggers. For example, if you're eliminating dairy, that means no milk, cheese, yogurt, or any products containing milk proteins.

STEP 3: THE CHALLENGE PHASE
After the elimination period, it's time to play Food Detective.

☞ Reintroduce one food group at a time, every 3–7 days.

☞ Start with a small amount and gradually increase.

☞ Carefully observe and record any symptoms.

☞ If symptoms occur, remove the food and wait until symptoms subside before introducing the next food.

A study in the *International Journal of Molecular Sciences* found that this systematic reintroduction approach can help identify specific food intolerances with up to 70% accuracy. That's some serious food sleuthing.

STEP 4: INTERPRET YOUR RESULTS

Now it's time to analyze your findings.

- ⮑ Search for patterns in your symptom diary.

- ⮑ Consider the timing and severity of symptoms.

- ⮑ Consult a healthcare professional to discuss your results.

- ⮑ Create a long-term plan based on your findings.

Remember, the goal isn't to restrict your diet forever, but to identify problematic foods and find a balanced approach that works for you.

REINTRODUCING FOODS AND INTERPRETING RESULTS: THE GRAND FOOD FINAL

Alright, food detectives, you've done the hard work of eliminating and reintroducing foods. Now, let's talk about how to make sense of all this information and what to do next.

TIMING IS EVERYTHING. When reintroducing foods, pay close attention to when symptoms appear.

- ⮑ IMMEDIATE REACTIONS (WITHIN 2 HOURS): More likely to be an allergy.

- ⮑ DELAYED REACTIONS (2-48 HOURS LATER): More likely to be an intolerance.

A study in the journal *Allergy* found that delayed reactions are more common with food intolerances, affecting up to 70% of those with non-allergic food hypersensitivity. It's like your body's way of sending you a delayed text message.

SEVERITY MATTERS. The severity of your symptoms can give you clues about the nature of your reaction.

෴ Mild symptoms (slight discomfort, minor bloating): Might be a sensitivity or mild intolerance.

෴ Moderate symptoms (significant discomfort, clear skin reactions): Could be a more severe intolerance or mild allergy.

෴ Severe symptoms (difficulty breathing, severe digestive distress): An allergy; seek medical attention immediately.

CONSIDER CROSS-REACTIVITY. Sometimes, foods that are botanically related can cause similar reactions. Here are some examples.

෴ If you react to birch pollen, you might also react to apples, carrots, or celery.

෴ If you're allergic to latex, you might react to bananas, avocados, or kiwis.

A review in the journal *Current Allergy and Asthma Reports* found that up to 50% of people with latex allergies may experience cross-reactivity with certain foods. It's like your immune system playing a game of "guilty by association".

THE DOSE RESPONSE. Some people can tolerate small amounts of a problematic food but react to larger quantities. This is especially common with food intolerances:

෴ Keep track of the amounts you consume during reintroduction.

෴ Try different serving sizes to find your personal threshold.

෴ Consider Other Factors. Remember, other factors can influence your reactions:

  o Stress levels

  o Hormonal changes

  o Concurrent illnesses

o   Combination of foods

A study in the journal *Neurogastroenterology & Motility* found that stress can exacerbate symptoms of food intolerance in up to 75% of people with irritable bowel syndrome. It's like your gut has stage fright.

THE ELIMINATION DIET IS NOT FOREVER

The goal of an elimination diet is to identify problem foods, not to restrict your diet indefinitely. Some people may need to avoid certain foods long-term (like those with severe allergies). Others might be able to reintroduce foods in small amounts or in less processed forms. Work with a healthcare provider or registered dietitian to develop a long-term plan.

A WORD OF CAUTION

When to seek professional help!

While elimination diets can be a powerful tool, they're not without risks.

- ⚡ NUTRITIONAL DEFICIENCIES: Eliminating multiple food groups can lead to nutrient gaps.

- ⚡ DISORDERED EATING PATTERNS: The restrictive nature of elimination diets can trigger disordered eating in susceptible individuals.

- ⚡ MISSING UNDERLYING CONDITIONS: Some symptoms might be caused by conditions unrelated to food.

Always consult a healthcare provider before starting an elimination diet, especially if:

↬ You suspect a severe food allergy.

↬ You have a history of eating disorders.

↬ You have multiple chronic health conditions. The same applies if you're pregnant or breastfeeding.

A study in the *Journal of the Academy of Nutrition and Dietetics* found that supervised elimination diets led to better outcomes and fewer nutritional deficiencies compared to self-directed elimination diets. Sometimes, two heads (yours and a professional's) are better than one.

SPECIAL CONSIDERATIONS FOR DIFFERENT AGE GROUPS

Food sensitivities can affect people of all ages, but there are some special considerations for different life stages.

INFANTS AND YOUNG CHILDREN

Food allergies are more common in children, with about 8% of children having at least one food allergy. The most common allergens in children are milk, eggs, and peanuts. Some children outgrow their allergies, especially to milk and eggs. A study in the journal *Pediatrics* found that introducing peanuts early (between 4 and 11 months) in high-risk infants significantly reduced the risk of developing peanut allergies. It's like giving your baby's immune system an early education.

ADOLESCENTS AND YOUNG ADULTS

New allergies can develop during puberty due to hormonal changes. Social pressures and a desire for independence can make managing food allergies challenging.

ADULTS

Adult-onset food allergies are less common but can occur. Hormonal changes (like pregnancy or menopause) can affect food sensitivities.

OLDER ADULTS

Changes in digestion and immune function can lead to new food intolerances. Medications can interact with certain foods, mimicking intolerance symptoms.

A study in the journal *Immunity & Aging* found that the prevalence of food intolerances increases with age, impacting up to 25% of older adults. It's like your body decides to become a picky eater in its golden years.

BRINGING IT ALL TOGETHER
YOUR FOOD SENSITIVITY ACTION PLAN

Alright, food sensitivity sleuths, ready to take control of your diet and feel better? Here's a simple action plan to get you started.

- **KEEP A FOOD AND SYMPTOM DIARY:** Start tracking what you eat and how you feel for at least two weeks.

- **IDENTIFY SUSPECT FOODS:** Based on your diary and common allergens, make a list of potential trigger foods.

- **PLAN YOUR ELIMINATION DIET:** Decide which foods to eliminate and for how long. Plan your meals accordingly.

- **CONDUCT THE ELIMINATION PHASE:** Remove suspect foods for 2-4 weeks, being vigilant about hidden sources.

- **REINTRODUCE FOODS SYSTEMATICALLY:** Bring back one food group at a time, carefully observing any reactions.

- **ANALYZE YOUR RESULTS:** Search for patterns in your reactions and consider the timing and severity of symptoms.

- **DEVELOP A LONG-TERM PLAN:** Work with a healthcare provider to create a balanced diet that avoids trigger foods but meets all your nutritional needs.

- **STAY FLEXIBLE:** Remember that food sensitivities can change over time. Be open to retesting foods in the future.

A Final Thought on Food Sensitivities and Elimination Diets

As we wrap up our deep dive into the world of food sensitivities and elimination diets, it's important to remember that our relationship with food is complex and deeply personal. What works for one person may not work for another, and that's okay.

The goal of exploring food sensitivities isn't to label foods as "good" or "bad," but to understand how different foods interact with your unique body. It's about empowering yourself with knowledge and finding a way of eating that helps you feel your best.

Remember, food is more than just fuel—it's a source of pleasure, cultural connection, and social bonding. If you find that certain foods don't agree with you, focus on all the delicious options that do make you feel good, rather than dwelling on what you can't eat.

And finally, always approach changes to your diet with curiosity, patience, and self-compassion. Your body is an incredible, complex system, and learning to listen to its signals is a lifelong journey.

Here's to happy eating, symptom-free living, and becoming the best food detective, you can be.

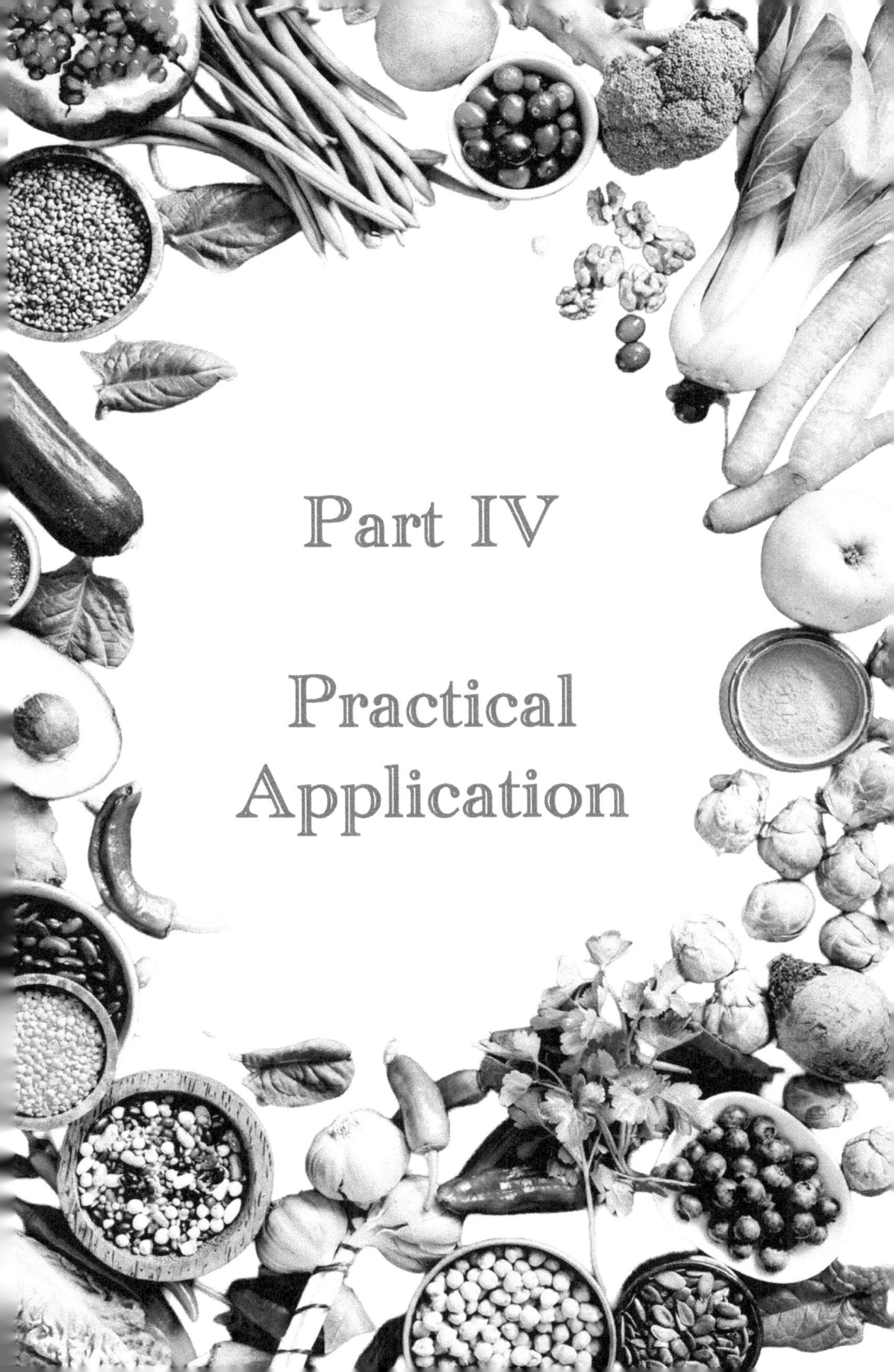

Part IV

Practical Application

CHAPTER 13

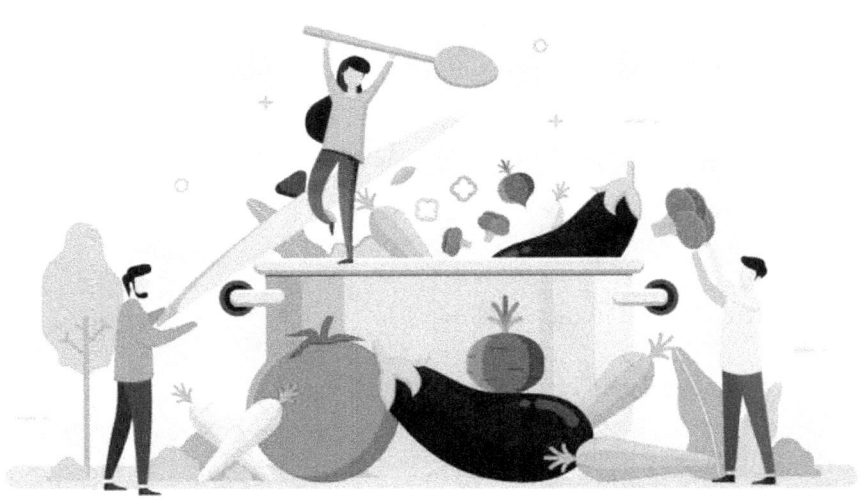

STOCKING A HEALING KITCHEN

YOUR HEALTH FOOD HEADQUARTERS

Kitchen commanders and pantry pioneers. You can turn your kitchen into a veritable fortress of health. We're going to transform that room where you occasionally burn toast into a superhero lair of nutritional goodness. So, put on your healthiest apron, and let's dive into creating a kitchen that would make even the most zealous nutritionist swoon.

ESSENTIAL INGREDIENTS
FOR A HEALTH-PROMOTING PANTRY
YOUR NUTRITIONAL A-TEAM

First things first, let's stock that pantry with some heavy hitters in the health department. These aren't just ingredients; they're your nutritional Special Forces team.

WHOLE GRAINS: THE COMPLEX CARB COMMANDOS

- Quinoa: The protein-packed pseudo-grain.

- Brown rice: The fiber-rich classic.

- Oats: The heart-healthy breakfast hero.

- Buckwheat: The gluten-free grain imposter (it's a seed).

PRO TIP: Store grains in airtight containers in a cool, dry place. They'll last longer and stay fresher, ready for action whenever you need them.

LEGUMES: THE PLANT-PROTEIN POWERHOUSE

- Lentils: Quick-cooking and versatile.

- Chickpeas: Hummus's main squeeze.

- Black Beans: The antioxidant all-star.

- Split Peas: The soup superstar.

FUN FACT: A study in the journal *Nutrients* found that regular legume consumption was associated with a 14% lower risk of developing type 2 diabetes. Take that, blood sugar spikes.

NUTS AND SEEDS: THE HEALTHY FAT TASK FORCE

- Almonds: The vitamin E virtuoso.

- Chia seeds: The omega-3 overachiever.

- Walnuts: The brain-boosting nut.

- Pumpkin seeds: The zinc zealot.

STORAGE TIP: Keep nuts and seeds in the fridge or freezer to prevent their healthy oils from going rancid. They'll stay fresh and crunchy for months.

HERBS AND SPICES: THE FLAVOR SWAT TEAM

- Turmeric: The anti-inflammatory icon.

- Cinnamon: The Blood Sugar Balancer.

- Garlic Powder: The Heart Health Hero.

- Oregano: The antioxidant.

ACE SPICE HACK: Buy whole spices when possible and grind them as needed. They'll stay potent longer, and your taste buds will thank you.

HEALTHY OILS: THE LIPID LIBERATION FRONT

- Extra Virgin Olive Oil: The Mediterranean diet superstar.

- Avocado Oil: The high-heat hero.

↗ Coconut Oil: The MCT maestro.

↗ Flaxseed Oil: The omega-3 champion (but don't heat it).

OIL WISDOM: Store oils away from light and heat to prevent oxidation. Your healthy fats will stay… well, healthy.

SUPERFOODS: THE NUTRITIONAL NAVY SEALS

↗ Spirulina: The protein-packed algae.

↗ Cacao Powder: The antioxidant-rich chocolate source.

↗ Goji Berries: The vision-supporting snack.

↗ Maca Powder: The energy-boosting root.

Remember, superfoods are great, but they're not magic bullets. Use them to enhance an already balanced diet, not as a replacement for whole foods.

CHOOSING AND STORING PRODUCE
FOR MAXIMUM NUTRITION
THE FRESH FOOD FRONTLINE

Now that we've got our pantry stocked, let's talk about keeping your fridge filled with nature's medicine cabinet: fruits and veggies.

THE CLEAN FIFTEEN AND DIRTY DOZEN
YOUR ORGANIC BUYING GUIDE

Not all produce needs to be organic. Save money by focusing on organic for the "Dirty Dozen" (foods with the most pesticide residues) and conventional for the "Clean Fifteen".

DIRTY DOZEN (GO ORGANIC)

- ☞ Strawberries

- ☞ Spinach

- ☞ Kale

- ☞ Nectarines

- ☞ Apples

CLEAN FIFTEEN (CONVENTIONAL IS OK)

- ☞ Avocados

- ☞ Sweet corn

- ☞ Pineapple

- ☞ Onions

- ☞ Papaya

<u>COLOR CODING</u>
EAT THE RAINBOW

Different colors in fruits and veggies represent different phytonutrients. Aim for a rainbow on your plate.

- ☞ RED: Lycopene (tomatoes, watermelon).

- ☞ ORANGE/ Beta-carotene (carrots, sweet potatoes).

- ☞ GREEN: Chlorophyll and isothiocyanates (broccoli, kale).

- ☞ BLUE/PURPLE: Anthocyanins (blueberries, eggplant).

139

⚡ WHITE: Allicin (garlic, onions).

PROPER STORAGE
KEEPING YOUR PRODUCE PERKY

⚡ Ethylene-producers (apples, bananas) should be stored separately from ethylene-sensitive foods (leafy greens, peppers).

⚡ Store herbs like a bouquet in water in the fridge.

⚡ Keep potatoes and onions in a cool, dark place—but not together.

PRO TIP: A study in the *Journal of Agricultural and Food Chemistry* found that storing cut lettuce in containers with a few apple slices can help keep it crisp longer due to the ethylene gas. It's like apples are the fountain of youth for lettuce.

KITCHEN TOOLS FOR HEALTHY COOKING
YOUR CULINARY ARSENAL

Alright, health food heroes, let's gear up with some kitchen gadgets that'll make healthy cooking a breeze.

HIGH-SPEED BLENDER: THE SMOOTHIE SORCERER
Perfect for making these foods.

⚡ Creamy smoothies.

⚡ Homemade nut butters.

⚡ Silky soups.

BLENDER HACK: Add leafy greens to your fruit smoothies for a nutrient boost without changing the taste much. Spinach in a strawberry banana smoothie? You'll never know it's there.

FOOD PROCESSOR: THE CHOPPING CHAMPION

Great for making these foods.

- ☞ Homemade energy balls.

- ☞ Quick-chopped veggies.

- ☞ Cauliflower "rice".

SPIRALIZER: THE NOODLE NINJA

Use it for making these foods.

- ☞ Zucchini noodles.

- ☞ Carrot ribbons.

- ☞ Sweet potato spirals.

SPIRALIZER TIP: Use it to make veggie "noodles" for a low-carb pasta alternative.

A study in the journal *Nutrients* found that replacing regular pasta with veggie noodles can significantly reduce calorie intake while increasing vegetable consumption. Noodle on that.

AIR FRYER: THE OIL-FREE ORCHESTRATOR

Perfect for making healthy versions of your favorite fried food!

- ☞ Crispy veggies.

- ☞ "Fried" chicken (without the frying).

- ☞ Roasted chickpeas.

INSTANT POT: THE ONE-POT WONDER

Great for making hearty meals!

- ⚐ Quick-cooking beans.

- ⚐ Tender meats.

- ⚐ One-pot meals.

INSTANT POT MAGIC: Use it to make bone broth in a fraction of the time. A study in the Journal of Nutritional Science found that bone broth can be a good source of collagen, which may support joint health.

CAST IRON SKILLET: THE HEAT-RETAINING HERO
Use it for creating a variety of delicious dishes.

- ⚐ Searing meats.

- ⚐ One-pan meals.

- ⚐ Adding a bit of iron to your diet (seriously).

IRON-CLAD FACT: Cooking in cast iron can increase the iron content of your food, especially acidic foods like tomato sauce. It's like getting a mini-iron supplement with your meal.

Chapter 14

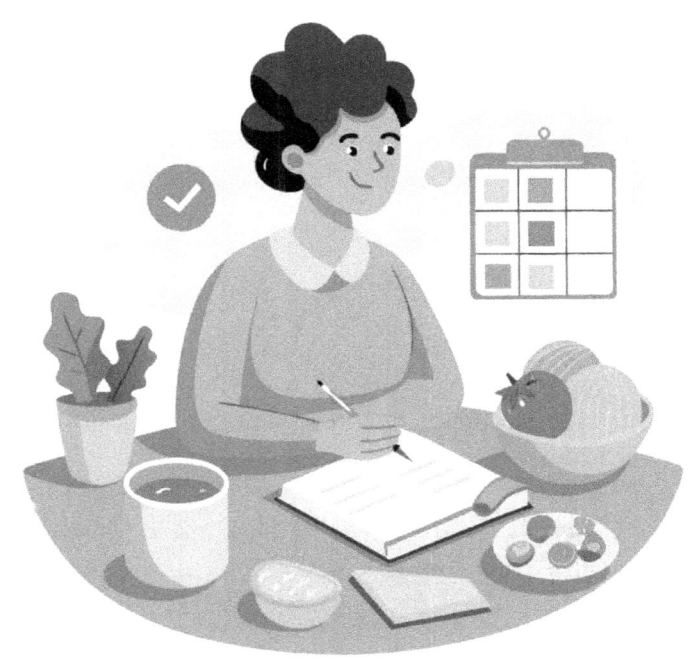

Meal Planning and Prep for Optimal Health

Your blueprint for nutritional success, meal prep maestros and planning prodigies. We turn all that beautiful, healthy food in your kitchen into actual meals. We're going to transform you from a "what's for dinner?" panic-googler to a meal-planning maven. Ready to become the architect of your nutritional destiny? Let's do this.

STRATEGIES FOR BALANCED MEAL PLANNING
YOUR DIETARY DESIGN PLAN

THE PLATE METHOD: YOUR MEAL-BUILDING BLUEPRINT
Think of your plate as a pie chart (mmm… pie).

- 1/2 Plate: Non-starchy vegetables.

- 1/4 Plate: Lean protein.

- 1/4 Plate: Complex carbs.

- Add a serving of healthy fats.

This simple visual guide helps ensure you're getting a good balance of nutrients at each meal.

THE 3-3-3 METHOD: YOUR WEEKLY MENU MATRIX
Plan for these three daily meals.

- 3 breakfast options.

- 3 lunch options.

- 3 dinner options.

MEAL PLANNING MAGIC: A study in the *American Journal of Preventive Medicine* found that meal planning was associated with a healthier diet and lower odds of obesity. It's like having a personal nutritionist in your pocket.

Rotate these throughout the week. This gives you variety without overwhelming you with options.

THEME NIGHTS: YOUR CULINARY CALENDAR
Assign themes to different nights of the week.

- ⚑ Meatless Monday.

- ⚑ Taco Tuesday.

- ⚑ Stir-Fry Friday.

This takes the guesswork out of "what's for dinner?" and can make grocery shopping easier.

PREP COMPONENTS, NOT FULL MEALS: YOUR MIX-AND-MATCH MEAL STRATEGY
Instead of preparing full meals, prep components that can be mixed and matched.

- ⚑ Grilled chicken.

- ⚑ Roasted veggies.

- ⚑ Cooked quinoa.

- ⚑ Homemade dressing.

This allows for more flexibility and prevents meal fatigue.

THE COLOR GAME: YOUR PRODUCE PURSUIT
Challenge yourself to include a certain number of different colored fruits and veggies each day. It's like playing nutritional bingo.

COLOR QUEST: A study in the *American Journal of Clinical Nutrition* found that a higher intake of different colored fruits and vegetables was associated with a lower risk of cognitive decline. Eat the rainbow to keep your brain sharp.

BATCH COOKING AND MEAL PREP TECHNIQUES
YOUR TIME-SAVING TACTICS

THE SUNDAY PREP POWER HOUR: YOUR WEEKLY KITCHEN KICKOFF

Dedicate an hour on Sunday (or whatever day works for you) to do meal prep.

- Wash and Chop Veggies.

- Cook a big batch of grains.

- Prepare a large protein (like a whole chicken or pot of beans).

THE SHEET PAN STRATEGY: YOUR ONE-PAN PLAN

- Roast a variety of vegetables on a sheet pan.

- Use different seasoning blends for variety.

- Add a protein source for a complete meal.

SHEET PAN SECRET: Lining your pan with parchment paper makes for easy cleanup and can reduce the need for added oils.

SOUP AND STEW STOCKPILE: YOUR LIQUID LUNCH (AND DINNER)

- Make a big batch of soup or stew.

- Portion into individual containers.

- Freeze for future meals.

SOUP SCIENCE: A study in the *British Journal of Nutrition* found that starting a meal with soup increased vegetable consumption and reduced calorie intake. Slurp your way to health.

Breakfast Batch Bonanza: Your Morning Meal Mastery

Prepare breakfast items in bulk.

- ☞ Overnight oats

- ☞ Egg muffins

- ☞ Chia seed pudding

Freezer Meal Frenzy: Your Future Food Stash

Prepare meals designed for freezing.

- ☞ Casseroles.

- ☞ Marinated meats.

- ☞ Homemade veggie burgers.

FREEZER FACT: Properly stored, most freezer meals can last 3-6 months. It's like sending a care package to your future self.

Salad Jar Jackpot: Your Layered Lunch Solution

Create salads in Mason jars.

- ☞ Dressing on the bottom.

- ☞ Hard veggies next.

- ☞ Proteins and softer veggies on top.

- ☞ Greens at the very top.

When you're ready to eat, just shake and enjoy.

BRINGING IT ALL TOGETHER
YOUR MEAL PLANNING AND PREP ACTION PLAN

Alright, kitchen warriors, ready to conquer meal planning and prep? Here's your battle plan.

STOCK YOUR ARSENAL
Fill your pantry and fridge with the essential ingredients we discussed.

PLAN YOUR ATTACK
Use the meal planning strategies to create a weekly menu. Remember the 3-3-3 method or theme nights to keep it simple and varied.

PREP YOUR WEAPONS
Dedicate time for batch cooking and meal prep. Even an hour on the weekend can set you up for success all week.

MIX AND MATCH
Prepare versatile components that can be combined in different ways throughout the week.

STORE SMART
Use proper food storage techniques to keep your prepped ingredients fresh and ready to use.

STAY FLEXIBLE
Remember, meal planning is a guide, not a strict rulebook. Be ready to adapt as needed.

EXPERIMENT WITH RECIPES
Try out different recipes tailored to your health goals. Don't be afraid to modify them to suit your tastes and nutritional needs.

A FINAL THOUGHT
ON PRACTICAL APPLICATION

As we wrap up our journey through the practical side of healthy eating, remember that creating a healing kitchen and mastering meal planning are skills that develop over time. Don't expect perfection right out of the gate. Like any new habit, it takes practice and patience to become second nature.

The goal isn't to create picture-perfect meals or stick to a rigid plan 100% of the time. Instead, focus on progress over perfection. Celebrate the small wins, like trying a new veggie or prepping your lunches for the week. These small steps add up to significant changes in your health and wellbeing.

Remember, your kitchen is more than just a place to prepare food. It's a laboratory for better health, a playground for culinary creativity, and a hub for nourishing not just your body but also your mind and spirit. By stocking your pantry with health-promoting foods, equipping yourself with the right tools, and arming yourself with smart meal planning strategies, you're setting the stage for a lifetime of better health.

So go forth, kitchen commanders. May your pantry be ever-stocked, your meal prep game strong, and your plates filled with colorful, nourishing foods. Here's to your health, one delicious, home-cooked meal at a time.

BONUS TIPS FOR MEAL PLANNING SUCCESS

Before we completely wrap up, let's throw in a few extra tips to really supercharge your meal planning and prep game.

THE LEFTOVER MAKEOVER: PLAN FOR INTENTIONAL LEFTOVERS

Cook extra of certain components to repurpose later in the week. Here are some ideas to get you started.

- ☞ Grilled chicken becomes chicken salad or goes into a stir-fry.

- ☞ Roasted vegetables get blended into a soup or added to a frittata.

- ☞ Cooked quinoa transforms into breakfast porridge or veggie burger base.

LEFTOVER MAGIC: A study in the *International Journal of Behavioral Nutrition and Physical Activity* found that cooking at home more often was associated with better diet quality and lower food expenses. Repurposing leftovers can help you cook at home more without feeling like you're always in the kitchen.

THE FLAVOR BOOSTER BANK: CREATE YOUR OWN SEASONING BLENDS

Mix up your seasoning blends to add instant flavor to simple meals.

- ☞ Taco seasoning.

- ☞ Italian herb blend.

- ☞ Curry powder.

- ☞ All-purpose savory seasoning.

SPICE IT UP: Herbs and spices aren't just flavor enhancers; they're nutritional powerhouses.

A review in the *Journal of AOAC International* found that many common herbs and spices have significant antioxidant properties.

THE SNACK ATTACK PLAN: PREP HEALTHY SNACKS

Don't forget to plan for snacks. Prep grab-and-go options.

- Cut veggies with homemade hummus.

- Trail mix with nuts and dried fruit.

- Hard-boiled eggs.

- Homemade energy balls.

SNACK FACT: A study in the *Journal of the American Dietetic Association* found that snackers had higher intakes of fruits, whole grains, and milk than non-snackers. It's all about choosing nutrient-dense options.

THE FROZEN ASSET: EMBRACE YOUR FREEZER

Your freezer is a meal prepper's best friend. Below are some freezer-friendly ideas.

- Smoothie Packs: Pre-portion smoothie ingredients in bags for easy blending.

- Cooked Grains: Freeze in portion-sized containers.

- Homemade Sauces and Pestos: Freeze in ice cube trays for easy portioning.

FREEZER WISDOM: Contrary to popular belief, freezing doesn't significantly decrease the nutritional value of foods. In fact, a study in the *Journal of Agricultural and Food Chemistry* found that frozen fruits and vegetables can have just as much, and sometimes more, nutrients than their fresh counterparts.

THE TECH SUPPORT: USE APPS AND TOOLS

Leverage technology to make meal planning easier.

- ☞ Meal planning apps for recipe storage and grocery list creation.

- ☞ Smart kitchen scales for easy portion control.

- ☞ Online grocery ordering for timesaving.

TECH TIDBIT: A study in the *Journal of Medical Internet Research* found that using a smartphone app for meal planning was associated with improved diet quality and increased fruit and vegetable intake.

THE SOCIAL SYNC: ALIGN YOUR MEAL PLAN WITH YOUR SOCIAL CALENDAR

Don't forget to account for social events, date nights, or busy evenings when meal planning. Plan for quick, easy meals on busy nights. Leave room for dining out or social events. Prepare extra on less busy days to cover for hectic ones.

BALANCING ACT: Remember, a healthy diet is one that's sustainable and enjoyable.

A study in the journal *Appetite* found that perceived difficulty in preparing healthy meals was a barrier to healthy eating. By planning around your lifestyle, you make healthy eating more achievable and less stressful.

And there you have it, health food heroes. You're now armed with a pantry full of nutritional superstars, a toolkit of meal planning strategies, and a repertoire of healthy recipes. Remember, the journey to optimal health through food is a marathon, not a sprint. Take it one meal at a time, and before you know it, you'll be a master of your own nutritional destiny.

Here's to your health, happiness, and many delicious meals to come.

CHAPTER 15

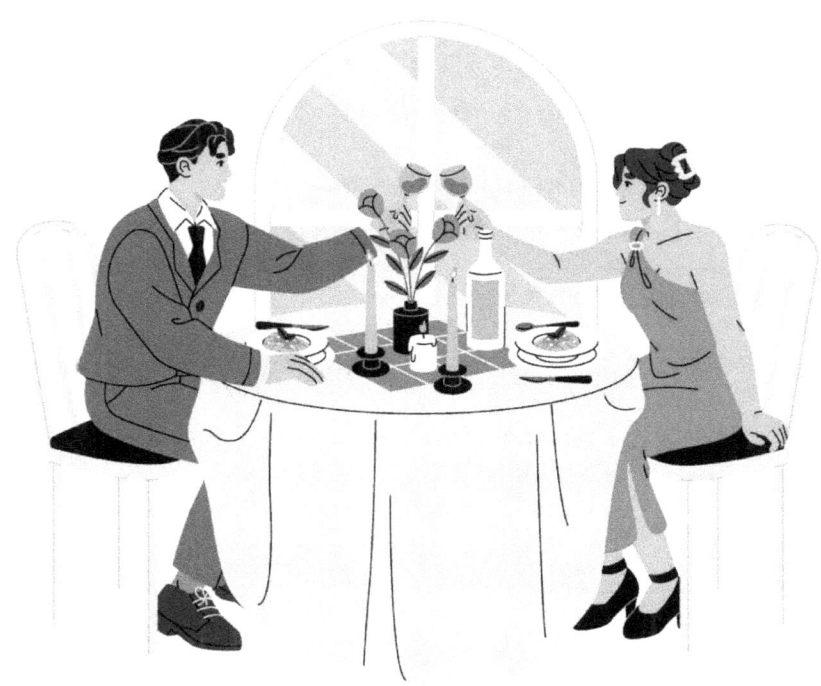

NAVIGATING EATING OUT AND SOCIAL SITUATIONS

STAYING HEALTHY IN THE WILD

The social butterflies and dining-out divas. It's time to tackle one of the most difficult challenges in maintaining a healthy diet: eating outside your carefully curated kitchen kingdom. Whether you're hitting up the hottest new restaurant or navigating Aunt Edna's annual potluck, we're going to arm you with strategies to keep your health goals on track without becoming a social pariah. So, put on your healthy eating armor, and let's dive into the wonderful world of dining out and socializing.

MAKING HEALTHY CHOICES AT RESTAURANTS
YOU'RE DINING OUT DEFENSIVE PLAYBOOK

THE MENU RECOGNITION MISSION
Before you even set foot in the restaurant, do some scouting.

- Check the menu online.

- Seek healthier options or dishes that can be easily modified.

- Have a game plan before you arrive.

MENU MASTERY: A study in the *Journal of Public Health* found that people who viewed menu information before dining out made healthier choices and consumed fewer calories. Knowledge is power, folks.

THE APPETIZER AMBUSH
Appetizers can be a minefield of hidden calories. Here's how to navigate the appetizer menu.

- Opt for broth-based soups or salads with dressing on the side.

- Share appetizers to control portion sizes.

- Beware of "healthy-sounding" options that may be high in calories (I'm looking at you, spinach and artichoke dip.)

APPETIZER INTEL: Research in the journal *Appetite* found that people who ordered a low-calorie appetizer ended up consuming fewer calories during their meal. Start light to finish right.

THE MAIN COURSE MANEUVER

When it comes to entrées, use these tactics.

- ⚑ Look for grilled, baked, or roasted options instead of fried.

- ⚑ Ask for sauces and dressings on the side.

- ⚑ Don't be afraid to ask for modifications (e.g., extra veggies instead of fries).

PORTION CONTROL PRO-TIP: Ask for a to-go box when your meal arrives and immediately pack up half. You'll have lunch for tomorrow and avoid overeating.

THE SNEAKY SIDES SITUATION

Side dishes can make or break your healthy meal. Here's the game plan.

- ⚑ Swap out fries or mashed potatoes for a side salad or steamed veggies.

- ⚑ If you're craving a less healthy side, share it with the table.

- ⚑ Be wary of "healthy" sides that might be doused in butter or oil.

SIDE DISH SCIENCE: A study in the *Journal of the Academy of Nutrition and Dietetics* found that increasing the portion size of vegetables on a plate led to increased vegetable consumption without increasing calorie intake. Size matters when it comes to veggies.

THE DESSERT DILEMMA

Ah, the sweet siren calls of the dessert menu. Here's how to handle it.

- ⚑ Share a dessert with the table.

- ⚑ Opt for fruit-based desserts.

↬ Consider ending your meal with a cup of tea or coffee instead.

SWEET STRATEGY: If you know you'll want dessert, plan for it by making lighter choices earlier in the meal. It's all about balance.

THE BEVERAGE BATTLEFIELD

Don't forget about liquid calories. Here's your drinking game plan.

↬ Water is always your best bet.

↬ If you're drinking alcohol, alternate with water.

↬ Beware of sugary cocktails and opt for wine, light beer, or spirits with low-calorie mixers.

DRINK WISDOM: A study in the *American Journal of Clinical Nutrition* found that people who drank water before and during a meal consumed fewer calories and reported feeling just as satisfied as those who didn't. Hydrate to dominate.

MAINTAINING DIETARY GOALS DURING SOCIAL EVENTS
YOUR PARTY-PROOF PLAN

THE PRE-PARTY PREP

Don't arrive at a social event starving. Try these pre-party tactics.

↬ Have a small, protein-rich snack before you go.

↬ Drink water to stay hydrated.

↬ Remind yourself of your health goals.

HUNGER HACK: Research in the *Journal of the American Dietetic Association* found that eating a small, high-protein snack before a meal can lead to reduced calorie intake. Snack smart to party smart.

THE BUFFET BATTLE PLAN

Facing down a buffet? Here's your strategy.

- ☞ Survey all options before filling your plate

- ☞ Start with veggies and lean proteins.

- ☞ Use a smaller plate to control portions.

BUFFET BRILLIANCE: A study in the journal *PLOS ONE* found that using a smaller plate at a buffet led to a 20% reduction in calorie consumption compared to using a larger plate. Size matters.

THE POTLUCK PREDICAMENT

When you're asked to bring a dish, seize the opportunity.

- ☞ Bring a healthy dish you know you can enjoy.

- ☞ Make it substantial enough to serve as your main meal if needed.

- ☞ Share the recipe—you might inspire others.

POTLUCK POWER MOVE: By bringing a healthy dish, you're not only ensuring you have something nutritious to eat, but you're also introducing others to tasty, healthy options. Be the change you want to see in the potluck world.

THE ALCOHOL ACTION PLAN

If you choose to drink, do it mindfully.

- ☞ Set a drink limit before you arrive.

- ☞ Opt for lower-calorie options like wine or spirits with soda water.

- ☞ Alternate alcoholic drinks with water.

SOBERING STAT: A study in the *American Journal of Clinical Nutrition* found that alcohol consumption before a meal increased calorie intake by 11%. Drink wisely.

THE MINDFUL MINGLING METHOD
Don't let socializing derail your healthy eating.

- Position yourself away from the food table.

- Focus on conversation rather than constant snacking.

- Keep your hands busy with a glass of water.

MINGLING MINDFULNESS: Research in the journal *Appetite* found that people consumed less food when they were engaged in a cognitively demanding task. So, dive deep into those conversations.

THE DAY-AFTER DEFENSE
If you do overindulge, don't let it derail you.

- Get back on track with your next meal.

- Squeeze in some extra movement the next day.

- Don't punish yourself; one indulgent event won't undo all your hard work.

BOUNCE-BACK WISDOM: A study in the *International Journal of Obesity* found that people who quickly got back on track after a dietary lapse were more successful in long-term weight management. It's not about perfection; it's about consistency.

COMMUNICATING DIETARY NEEDS TO OTHERS
YOUR DIPLOMATIC DINING DIALOGUE

THE HOST HELPER
Here's a good guide for when you're invited to someone's home.

- Offer to bring a dish that fits your dietary needs.

↪ Communicate your dietary restrictions well in advance.

↪ Express gratitude for their understanding and accommodations.

HOST HINT: A study in the *Journal of Nutrition Education and Behavior* found that people were more likely to try unfamiliar healthy foods when they were prepared by friends or family. Your healthy dish might be a hit.

THE RESTAURANT REQUESTOR

When dining out with others:

↪ Suggest restaurants that can accommodate various dietary needs.

↪ Don't be afraid to ask the server for modifications.

↪ Frame your choices positively (e.g., "I'm excited to try their grilled salmon", rather than "I can't eat anything fried").

RESTAURANT REALITY: Many restaurants are happy to accommodate dietary requests. A survey by the *National Restaurant Association* found that 93% of restaurants offer menu items for customers with food allergies.

THE WORKPLACE WARRIOR

Navigating work events and office treats.

↪ Keep healthy snacks at your desk to avoid temptation.

↪ Suggest healthier options for office celebrations.

↪ Lead by example with your food choices.

OFFICE INSIGHT: A study in the *American Journal of Health Promotion* found that workplace wellness programs that included healthy eating initiatives led to improved dietary behaviors among employees. Be the change in your office.

THE FAMILY FEAST FACILITATOR
Here's how to deal with family gatherings and traditions.

- Offer to help with meal planning and preparation.

- Introduce new, healthier versions of family favorites.

- Share the reasons behind your dietary choices (focus on how you feel, not on weight).

Research in the *Journal of Nutrition Education and Behavior* found that family members' eating habits significantly influence each other. Your healthy choices could have a ripple effect.

THE SOCIAL MEDIA SAVVY
Use social media to support your dietary goals.

- Share your healthy meals and recipes.

- Join online communities focused on your dietary approach.

- Use social media to find restaurants and recipes that align with your goals.

SOCIAL MEDIA STRATEGY: A study in the *Journal of Medical Internet Research* found that social media support was associated with greater weight loss success. Your Instagram food pics might be more than just pretty—they could be motivating you and others.

THE CONFIDENT COMMUNICATOR
Remember, you don't owe anyone an explanation for your food choices, but if you choose to share:

- Be positive and focus on how your diet makes you feel.

- Avoid preaching or trying to convert others.

- Express appreciation for others' understanding and support.

COMMUNICATION CLARITY: Research in the journal *Health Communication* found that positive, non-judgmental communication about dietary choices was more effective in influencing others' behaviors than negative or preachy approaches. Honey catches more flies than vinegar.

Bringing It All Together
Your Social Eating Success Plan

Alright, social butterflies, ready to spread your healthy eating wings? Here's your action plan for navigating eating out and social situations.

Plan
Whether it's checking restaurant menus or bringing a dish to a potluck, preparation is key.

Practice Portion Control
Use strategies like sharing dishes or using smaller plates to keep portions in check.

Make Smart Swaps
Seek opportunities to make healthy substitutions, like veggies instead of fries.

Stay Hydrated
Water is your best friend for controlling hunger and avoiding excess calories.

Mindful Indulgence
It's okay to enjoy treats occasionally. When you do, savor them fully and get back on track with your next meal.

Communicate Clearly
Don't be afraid to express your dietary needs but do so with positivity and gratitude.

Lead by Example
Your healthy choices might inspire others around you.

Focus on Fun
Remember, social events are about more than just food. Enjoy the company and activities.

A FINAL THOUGHT
ON NAVIGATING SOCIAL EATING

As we wrap up our guide to eating out and socializing, remember that food is just one part of these experiences. The joy of sharing a meal with friends, celebrating special occasions, or trying new cuisines is an important part of a balanced, happy life.

Your dietary choices are personal and important, but they don't have to define your social life. With the strategies we've discussed, you can maintain your health goals while still fully participating in social events and enjoying dining out.

Remember, it's all about balance and making choices that align with your overall health and happiness. Some days you might choose the salad, other days you might go for the burger—and both are okay. What matters is your basic pattern of eating and the joy you find in both your food and your social connections.

So go forth, social butterflies. May your restaurant choices be healthy, your potluck contributions be appreciated, and your social calendar be full. Here's to navigating the world of social eating with confidence, grace, and a side of veggies.

CHAPTER 16

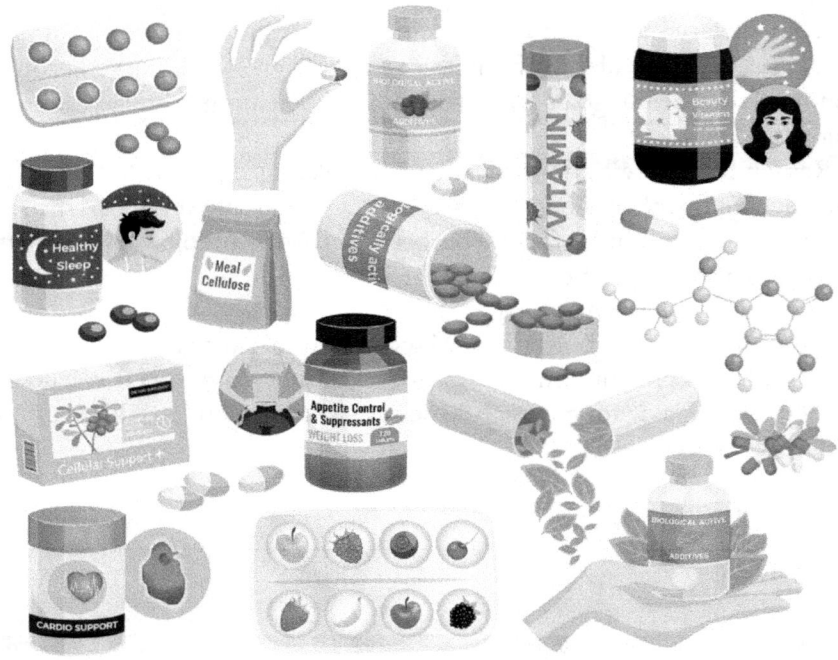

SUPPLEMENTS

WHEN AND HOW TO USE THEM

SEPARATING THE HELPERS FROM THE HYPE

Supplement sleuths and vitamin virtuosos. We will navigate the often confusing and sometimes controversial world of dietary supplements. With shelves upon shelves of colorful bottles promising everything from better sleep to superhuman strength, how do we separate the truly beneficial from the merely expensive urine producers? Buckle up because we're about to embark on a fact-filled journey through the supplement aisle.

EVALUATING SUPPLEMENT QUALITY AND SAFETY
YOUR SUPPLEMENT SHERLOCK TOOLKIT

Before we dive into specific supplements, let's talk about how to evaluate the quality and safety of any supplement you're considering.

LOOK FOR THIRD-PARTY TESTING
Reputable supplement companies typically have their products tested by independent third-party organizations. Look for seals from these organizations.

- USP (United States Pharmacopeia).

- NSF International.

- ConsumerLab.com.

QUALITY CONTROL FACT: A study published in *JAMA Network Open* found that 776 dietary supplements contained unapproved pharmaceutical ingredients. Third-party testing can help ensure you're getting what's on the label and nothing else.

These organizations test supplements for purity, potency, and contaminants.

CHECK FOR GMP CERTIFICATION
GMP stands for Good Manufacturing Practices. Look for supplements

made in GMP-certified facilities.

READ THE INGREDIENT LIST

Avoid supplements with unnecessary fillers, artificial colors, or allergens you're sensitive to.

CONSIDER THE FORM

Some forms of supplements are more easily absorbed than others. For example:

- ☞ Magnesium glycinate is typically better absorbed than magnesium oxide.

- ☞ Methyl cobalamin (a form of B12) is typically more bioavailable than cyanocobalamin.

ABSORPTION ACTION: A study in the *Journal of the American College of Nutrition* found that magnesium glycinate had superior absorption compared to magnesium oxide in human subjects.

BE WARY OF OUTRAGEOUS CLAIMS

If it sounds too good to be true, it is. Supplements can support health, but they're not magic pills.

Now, let's dive into some supplements with solid scientific backing for various health conditions.

ESSENTIAL SUPPLEMENTS
FOR DIFFERENT HEALTH CONDITIONS
THE SCIENCE-BACKED SUPERSTARS

OMEGA-3 FATTY ACIDS: THE HEART AND BRAIN BOOSTER

WHAT IT DOES
Supports heart health, brain function, and reduces inflammation.

THE SCIENCE

A meta-analysis published in the *Journal of the American Heart Association* found that omega-3 supplementation was associated with reduced risk of coronary heart disease and heart attack.

WHO MIGHT BENEFIT

- People with high triglycerides.

- Those at risk for heart disease.

- Individuals looking to support brain health.

DOSAGE

Typically, 250-500 mg combined EPA and DHA daily.

PRO TIP

Look for fish oil supplements that have been molecularly distilled to remove contaminants.

VITAMIN D: THE SUNSHINE SUPPLEMENT

WHAT IT DOES

Supports bone health, immune function, and mood.

THE SCIENCE

A systematic review in the *BMJ* found that vitamin D supplementation protected against acute respiratory tract infections, particularly in those who were very deficient.

WHO MIGHT BENEFIT

- People with limited sun exposure.

- Older adults.

- Those with dark skin.

🐦 Individuals with malabsorption issues.

DOSAGE

Varies widely based on individual needs. The RDA is 600–800 IU, but many experts recommend higher doses. Always consult a healthcare provider for personalized dosing.

VITAMIN D INSIGHT

A study in the *New England Journal of Medicine* found that vitamin D supplementation reduced the risk of fractures in older adults when combined with calcium.

PROBIOTICS: THE GUT HEALTH GUARDIANS

WHAT THEY DO

Support digestive health, immune function, and potentially mental health.

THE SCIENCE

A meta-analysis in the *World Journal of Gastroenterology* found that probiotics were effective in treating and preventing antibiotic-associated diarrhea.

WHO MIGHT BENEFIT

🐦 People with digestive issues.

🐦 Those taking antibiotics.

🐦 Individuals looking to support immune health.

DOSAGE

Varies by strain. Look for supplements with at least 1 billion CFUs (colony-forming units).

PROBIOTIC PARTICULARS

Not all probiotic strains are created equal. Different strains have different effects. For example, Lactobacillus rhamnosus GG has been well studied for preventing antibiotic-associated diarrhea.

MAGNESIUM: THE RELAXATION MINERAL

WHAT IT DOES
Supports muscle and nerve function, energy production, and sleep.

THE SCIENCE
A systematic review in the journal *Nutrients* found that magnesium supplementation significantly reduced blood pressure in individuals with insulin resistance, prediabetes, or other noncommunicable chronic diseases.

WHO MIGHT BENEFIT

- People with muscle cramps or tension.

- Those with sleep issues.

- Individuals with high blood pressure.

DOSAGE
The RDA is 310-420 mg for adults, depending on age and sex.

MAGNESIUM MAGIC
A study in the *Journal of Research in Medical Sciences* found that magnesium supplementation improved sleep efficiency, sleep time, and sleep onset latency in elderly individuals with insomnia.

VITAMIN B12: THE ENERGY ENHANCER

WHAT IT DOES
Supports energy production, nerve function, and red blood cell formation.

THE SCIENCE

A study in the *American Journal of Clinical Nutrition* found that vitamin B12 supplementation improved neurological symptoms in individuals with B12 deficiency.

WHO MIGHT BENEFIT

- ⚐ Vegetarians and vegans.

- ⚐ Older adults.

- ⚐ People with absorption issues.

- ⚐ Those with fatigue or neurological symptoms.

DOSAGE

The RDA is 2.4 mcg for adults, but higher doses are often used to treat deficiency.

B12 BOMBSHELL

A study in *Neurology* found that having vitamin B12 levels in the low-normal range was associated with an increased risk of accelerated cognitive decline and dementia in older adults.

ZINC: THE IMMUNE SYSTEM ALLY

WHAT IT DOES

Supports immune function, wound healing, and protein synthesis.

THE SCIENCE

A meta-analysis in the *Journal of the American Medical Association* found that zinc lozenges reduced the duration of the common cold when taken within 24 hours of symptom onset.

WHO MIGHT BENEFIT

- ⚐ People looking to support immune function.

🐾 Those with wound healing issues.

🐾 Individuals with taste or smell disorders.

DOSAGE
The RDA is 8–11 mg for adults, depending on sex.

ZINC ZINGER
While zinc can be beneficial, too much can be harmful. A study in the *British Journal of Clinical Pharmacology* found that excessive zinc intake can impair immune function and interfere with copper absorption.

IRON: THE OXYGEN TRANSPORTER

WHAT IT DOES
Essential for red blood cell production and oxygen transport.

THE SCIENCE
A systematic review in the *Cochrane Database of Systematic Reviews* found that daily iron supplementation effectively reduces iron deficiency anemia and improves hemoglobin concentrations.

WHO MIGHT BENEFIT

🐾 Menstruating women.

🐾 Pregnant women.

🐾 Vegetarians and vegans.

🐾 Endurance athletes.

DOSAGE
Varies widely based on individual needs. *Always consult a healthcare provider before starting iron supplementation.*

IRON INSIGHT

While iron is crucial for many bodily functions, too much can be harmful. A study in the *Journal of Clinical Investigation* found that excess iron can increase oxidative stress and inflammation.

CALCIUM: THE BONE BUILDER

WHAT IT DOES

Essential for bone health, muscle function, and nerve signaling.

THE SCIENCE

A meta-analysis in the *British Medical Journal* found that calcium supplementation reduced the risk of fractures, particularly in older individuals.

WHO MIGHT BENEFIT

- Postmenopausal women.

- Individuals with low dairy intake.

- Those at risk for osteoporosis.

DOSAGE

The RDA is 1000–1200 mg for adults, depending on age and sex.

CALCIUM CAUTION

While calcium is important for bone health, excessive supplementation may have risks. A study in the *Journal of the American Heart Association* found that calcium supplements were associated with an increased risk of coronary artery calcification.

VITAMIN C: THE ANTIOXIDANT ACE

WHAT IT DOES

Supports immune function, acts as an antioxidant, and aids in collagen production.

THE SCIENCE

A meta-analysis in the *European Journal of Clinical Nutrition* found that vitamin C supplementation reduced the duration of common cold symptoms.

WHO MIGHT BENEFIT

- Smokers (who have higher vitamin C requirements).

- People under high stress.

- Those looking to support skin health.

DOSAGE

The RDA is 65-90 mg for adults, but higher doses are often used.

VITAMIN C VERDICT

While vitamin C is safe, megadoses aren't necessary. A study in *JAMA Internal Medicine* found that high-dose vitamin C supplementation didn't reduce the incidence of colds in the general population.

POTENTIAL INTERACTIONS
BETWEEN SUPPLEMENTS AND MEDICATIONS
THE SUPPLEMENT SAFETY DANCE

While supplements can be beneficial, they can also interact with medications. Here are some important interactions to be aware of.

ST. JOHN'S WORT

This herb can interact with many medications, including antidepressants, birth control pills, and blood thinners. It can reduce the effectiveness of these medications.

VITAMIN K

Can interfere with blood-thinning medications like warfarin. If you're on blood thinners, maintain a consistent vitamin K intake and inform your doctor of any changes.

GINKGO BILOBA

Can increase the risk of bleeding when taken with blood thinners or NSAIDs.

IRON

Can reduce the absorption of certain antibiotics and thyroid medications. Take iron supplements at least two hours apart from these medications.

CALCIUM

Can interfere with the absorption of certain antibiotics and thyroid medications. Like iron, take calcium supplements at least two hours apart from these medications.

MAGNESIUM

Can interfere with the absorption of certain antibiotics and reduce the effectiveness of some medications for osteoporosis.

ZINC

High doses can reduce the absorption of certain antibiotics.

INTERACTION INSIGHT

A study in the Journal of the *American Medical Association* found that about 15% of older adults were at risk for a major drug-supplement interaction. Always inform your healthcare provider about all supplements you're taking.

Bringing It All Together
Your Supplement Success Strategy

Alright, supplement savants, ready to navigate the vitamin aisle with confidence? Here's your action plan.

Assess Your Needs
Consider your diet, lifestyle, and any health conditions you have.

Consult a Professional
Talk to your healthcare provider or a registered dietitian about which supplements might benefit you.

Quality Control
Choose supplements from reputable brands with third-party testing.

Start Low and Go Slow
Begin with the lowest effective dose and increase gradually if needed.

Monitor Your Response
Pay attention to how you feel and any changes in your health.

Regular Review
Reassess your supplement regimen periodically, as your needs may change over time.

Food First
Remember that supplements are meant to supplement, not replace, a healthy diet.

Drug Interactions
Always inform your healthcare provider about all supplements you're taking, especially if you're on medications.

A Final Thought
on Supplements

As we conclude our journey through the supplement aisle, it's important to remember that while supplements can play a valuable role in supporting health, they're not a magic bullet. The foundation of good health is still a balanced diet, regular exercise, adequate sleep, and stress management.

Supplements, when chosen wisely and used appropriately, can help fill nutritional gaps and support your health. However, they should be considered part of a holistic approach to health, not as a replacement for healthy lifestyle habits.

Remember, what works for one person may not work for another. Our nutritional needs are as individual as our fingerprints, influenced by our genes, lifestyle, environment, and health status. That's why it's crucial to work with healthcare professionals to develop a supplementation plan tailored to your unique needs.

Lastly, stay informed and critical. The world of nutrition science is constantly evolving, and new research emerges all the time. What we believe to be true about supplements today may change with future studies. Keep an open mind, stay curious, and always prioritize evidence-based information.

So, here's to smart supplementation, informed choices, and optimal health. May your vitamins be effective, your minerals well-absorbed, and your health ever improve.

CONCLUSION
FOOD AS FUEL—NOURISHING YOUR BODY, MIND, AND LIFE

Throughout this journey, we've explored the profound impact that food has on every aspect of our health and well-being. From the cellular level to our quality of life, the foods we choose to eat play a crucial role in shaping our health, performance, and longevity.

We began by delving into the foundations of food as medicine and fuel, exploring the science behind how nutrients interact with our bodies. We learned that food is not just calories but information—sending signals to our genes, influencing our gut microbiome, and affecting our brain chemistry.

We then embarked on a tour of how food can be used to address specific health conditions. We discovered how certain dietary approaches can support heart health, boost brain function, manage chronic pain, and enhance our immune system. We learned that food can be a powerful tool in preventing and managing a wide range of health issues, from diabetes to depression.

Our exploration then took us into the world of therapeutic diets and approaches. We examined the potential benefits and considerations of plant-based eating, ketogenic diets, and intermittent fasting. We learned that while there's no one-size-fits-all approach to nutrition, these dietary strategies can offer significant health benefits when applied appropriately.

We then rolled up our sleeves and got practical, learning how to stock a healing kitchen, plan, and prep meals for optimal health, and navigate the challenges of eating out and social situations. We discovered that with the right strategies, it's possible to keep a healthy diet in any setting.

Finally, we explored the world of supplements, learning when they can be beneficial and how to choose them wisely. We discovered that while supplements can play a valuable role in filling nutritional gaps, they're most effective when used as part of a comprehensive approach to health that prioritizes whole foods.

Throughout this book, one message has remained constant: food is the fuel that powers every function in our body. The quality of this fuel dramatically affects how well our 'engine' runs. By selecting nutrient-dense, whole foods, we provide our bodies with the premium fuel it needs to perform at its best.

But beyond just fuel, food is a source of pleasure, a centerpiece of social connection, and a powerful expression of culture and tradition. By understanding the impact of our food choices, we can create a relationship with food that nourishes not just our bodies but our whole selves.

Remember, the journey to optimal health through nutrition is just that—a journey. It's not about perfection, but about making informed choices more often than not. Small, consistent changes can lead to significant improvements in health over time.

As you move forward from here, I encourage you to stay curious, keep learning, and most importantly, listen to your body. Your nutritional needs are unique to you and may change over time. Be willing to experiment, adjust, and find what works best for you.

Thank you for joining me on this exploration of food as medicine and fuel. By picking up this book, you've taken an important step towards taking control of your health through the power of nutrition. I hope the information, strategies, and recipes we've shared will empower you to make choices that support your health and enhance your life.

Remember, every meal is an opportunity to nourish your body and invest in your health. Here's to your journey towards vibrant health, one delicious, nutritious bite at a time.

Thank you for reading, and here's to your health.

ABOUT THE AUTHOR

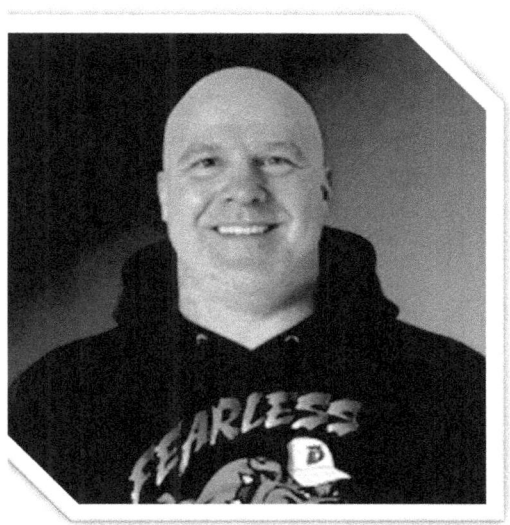

KEVIN B. DIBACCO

Kevin's life story is a powerful testament to the resilience of the human spirit. As a writer, Kevin draws from his experiences to share invaluable lessons on overcoming adversity and the temptation to quit. His words carry the weight of someone who has faced unimaginable challenges and emerged stronger, wiser, and more compassionate.

From a young age, Kevin's health struggles began, and he found himself facing one medical battle after another. By his 30s, he had endured a staggering 10 major medical procedures, including multiple knee operations, back surgeries, hip replacements, and treatment for an aggressive brain tumor. Even as he was writing his book, Kevin was struck by COVID-19, which led to pneumonia and daily nebulizer treatments. Lesser men might have given up, but Kevin refused to see himself as a victim of circumstance.

Through each diagnosis and rehabilitation, Kevin made a conscious choice to reframe adversity as an opportunity for growth. He focused on the small wins, visualizing himself healed and happy, and leaning on his deep faith and the support of loved ones during the darkest times. When fear or hopelessness crept in, he turned to prayer, uplifting books, and encouraging sayings to find the strength to take the next step forward.

As he navigated his journey, Kevin discovered the transformative power of the mind and positive thinking. He realized that by controlling his inner world—his thoughts, beliefs, and visualizations—he could shape his outer reality. This profound insight became the foundation for his book, in which he shares his medical battles alongside the techniques he used to stay grounded in positivity.

Kevin's book is not a theoretical exploration of resilience; it is a deeply personal account of his struggles and triumphs. He provides practical exercises to help readers overcome negative self-talk, face their fears, and visualize their desired outcomes. His message is one of hope and empowerment: regardless of what life throws at us, we have the power to choose our response.

Through his writing, Kevin aims to inspire others facing their battles to tap into their inner reserves of strength. He believes that by reframing difficulties as opportunities for growth and committing to personal development, we can overcome any obstacle, including those within our minds.

Kevin's story is a shining example of the human capacity for resilience and the power of the human spirit. His words serve as a reminder that, no matter how many times we are knocked down, we always have the choice to get back up. In sharing his journey, Kevin hopes to inspire others to keep going, even in the face of insurmountable odds.

Introduction: Food as Your Secret Weapon for Health and Performance

Hey there! Welcome to "Eat To Heal: A Practical Guide to Nourishing Your Body and Treating Disease Through Food.

" I'm thrilled you've picked up this book, and I can't wait to share with you the incredible power of food to transform your health, boost your performance, and even change your life.

Now, you might be wondering, "Who's this person, and why should I listen to him about food and health?" Well, allow me to introduce myself. I've been an athlete since I could walk. From Little League to high school sports, I've always been drawn to the thrill of competition and the satisfaction of pushing my body to its limits. But it wasn't until I discovered powerlifting and bodybuilding that I really found my groove.

Picture this: a chubby kid who could barely bench press the bar, transforming into a competitive powerlifter who could deadlift more than twice his body weight. Yeah, that was me. And let me tell you, that journey taught me a thing or two about the importance of what you put into your body.

I remember my first powerlifting meet like it was yesterday. I was nervous as hell, my palms sweating as I approached the platform. But as soon as I wrapped my hands around that bar, something clicked. The months of training, the careful attention to nutrition—it all came together in that moment. When I successfully lifted that weight, setting a personal record, I knew I was hooked.

As a competitive powerlifter, I quickly learned that food wasn't just fuel—it was the foundation of my performance. The right nutrition could mean the difference between setting a new personal record and falling short. And as I transitioned into bodybuilding and eventually became a trainer, I saw firsthand how dramatically the right (or wrong) food choices could impact not just performance but health and well-being.

But here's the kicker: despite being immersed in the world of fitness and nutrition, I still had a lot to learn about food as medicine. Sure, I knew all about protein shakes and carb-loading, but the idea that food could heal the body? That was a game-changer for me.

My "aha" moment came when I was dealing with some nagging injuries and inflammation that just wouldn't quit, no matter how much I stretched or how many ice baths I took. A nutritionist friend suggested I investigate anti-inflammatory foods, and, skeptical but desperate, I gave it a shot. Lo and behold, within a few weeks of tweaking my diet, I noticed a significant improvement. My recovery time shortened, my energy levels shot up, and I even started sleeping better.

That experience opened my eyes to the healing power of food, and I've been on a mission ever since to learn everything I can about using nutrition to optimize health and performance. And let me tell you, it's been one heck of a ride.

Follow my latest releases at these websites!

https://kbd.allauthor.com

www.ptbooksinc.com

BOOKS BY KEVIN DiBACCO

100 Unhealthy Foods

Back Care Made Easy: Simple Stretches and Exercises for Everyone

Bad Air: What Are We Breathing?

Badge of Horror

Being Weird: Unleash Your Inner Weirdo and Conquer the World

Chemicals in Our Food: What's Really on Your Plate?

Coffee: The Magic Brew

Dare to Believe: Building Unshakeable Confidence in All You Do

Desk Duty Fitness

Fitness Decoded: Unlocking the Secrets to Healthiness and Happiness at Any Age!

From Doubt to Believing: Removing the Doubt Obstacle in Our Life

Grip Strength: An Indicator of Your Overall Health

History and Evolution of Weightlifting and Equipment

Hold the Power

Hug It Out: Healing Through Hugging

Hysometrics

Hysterical Strength: The Extraordinary Display of Super Human Strength

Talk Yourself Into Greatness

Tea: The Mythical Beginnings

The Artist Sales Kit

The Confident Warrior: How to Cultivate Confidence in Everyday Life, Then Use It!

The Gabardine Gang: Power and Betrayal in Hartford's Mob

The Great Dimming: The Modern IQ Decline

The Handshake Around the World

The Lost Art of Logical Thinking

The Mozart Mind Effect

The Real World Guide to Digital Filmmaking

They Said What? Some of the Worst Predictions Ever Made!

The Symphony of the Soul: Classical Music and the Impact on Our Mood

Understanding and Overcoming Depression

Unsafe at Any Dose

Unstoppable: Success Through Persistence

We All Need Hope: Where There's Hope, There's a Way Forward

What is the Happiest Country on Earth?

Your Body Recipe: A Captivating Look at What Makes Us Human

FILMS BY KEVIN DIBACCO

Dark Minds (Sci-Fi Thriller)

Early Grave (Horror; Suspense)

APPENDIX A

HEALTHY RECIPES

HEALTHY RECIPES FOR VARIOUS HEALTH GOALS
YOUR CUSTOMIZED COOKBOOK

Now, let's put all this planning and prepping into action with some recipes tailored to different health goals.

Cauliflower Fried "Rice"
(For Weight Management)

Ingredients
- 4 cups cauliflower rice (pulse cauliflower in a food processor)
- 1 cup mixed vegetables (peas, carrots, bell peppers)
- 2 eggs, beaten
- 2 tbsp low-sodium soy sauce
- 1 tbsp sesame oil
- 2 cloves garlic, minced
- 1 inch ginger, grated

Instructions
1. Sauté garlic and ginger in sesame oil.
2. Add vegetables and cook until tender.
3. Push veggies to the side and scramble eggs in the pan.
4. Add cauliflower rice and soy sauce and stir-fry until heated through.

CALORIE-CUTTING TIP: This recipe swaps high-carb rice for low-calorie cauliflower, significantly reducing the calorie content while boosting the vegetable intake.

A study in the *European Journal of Clinical Nutrition* found that replacing rice with cauliflower rice led to a significant reduction in calorie and carbohydrate intake without affecting satiety.

MEDITERRANEAN QUINOA BOWL
(FOR HEART HEALTH)

INGREDIENTS
- 1 cup cooked quinoa
- 1/4 cup chickpeas
- 1/4 avocado, sliced
- 1/4 cup cherry tomatoes, halved
- 1/4 cup cucumber, diced
- 2 tbsp feta cheese
- 1 tablespoon olive oil
- 1 tsp lemon juice
- Fresh herbs (parsley, mint)

INSTRUCTIONS
1. Combine all ingredients in a bowl.
2. Drizzle with olive oil and lemon juice.
3. Toss and enjoy.

HEART-HEALTHY HINT: The combination of whole grains, legumes, and healthy fats in this bowl is a cardiovascular powerhouse.

A study in the *New England Journal of Medicine* found that a Mediterranean-style diet supplemented with extra-virgin olive oil or nuts reduced the risk of major cardiovascular events.

OMEGA-3 RICH SALMON SALAD
(FOR BRAIN HEALTH)

INGREDIENTS
- 4 oz cooked salmon, flaked
- 2 cups mixed greens
- 1/4 cup walnuts
- 1/4 cup blueberries
- 1/4 avocado, sliced
- 2 tbsp olive oil
- 1 tbsp balsamic vinegar

INSTRUCTIONS
1. Arrange greens on a plate.
2. Top with salmon, walnuts, blueberries, and avocado.
3. Drizzle with olive oil and balsamic vinegar.

BRAIN-BOOSTING BONUS: This salad is packed with omega-3 fatty acids from salmon and walnuts and antioxidants from blueberries.

A study in the journal *Neurology* found that higher levels of omega-3 fatty acids were associated with better brain structure and cognitive function.

PROBIOTIC POWERHOUSE SMOOTHIE
(FOR GUT HEALTH)

INGREDIENTS
- 1 cup unsweetened kefir
- 1 banana
- 1 cup spinach
- 1 tbsp chia seeds
- 1/2 cup blueberries
- 1 tsp. honey (optional)

INSTRUCTIONS
1. Blend all ingredients until smooth.
2. Enjoy immediately.

GUT-FRIENDLY FACT: This smoothie combines probiotics (from kefir) with prebiotics (from banana and chia seeds) to support a healthy gut microbiome.

A study in the journal *Nutrients* found that consuming both prebiotics and probiotics (known as synbiotics) had greater benefits for gut health than consuming either alone.

TURMERIC GINGER IMMUNE-BOOSTING SOUP
(FOR IMMUNE SUPPORT)

INGREDIENTS:
- 4 cups vegetable broth
- 1 can coconut milk
- 1 tablespoon grated ginger. 1 tablespoon turmeric
- 2 cloves garlic, minced
- 1 cup mixed vegetables (carrots, celery, onions)
- 1 cup cooked chicken or tofu
- Juice of 1 lemon
- Salt and pepper to taste

INSTRUCTIONS:
1. Sauté vegetables, garlic, ginger, and turmeric in a pot.
2. Add broth and coconut milk; simmer for 15 minutes.
3. Add chicken or tofu and lemon juice; heat through.
4. Season with salt and pepper.

IMMUNE-BOOSTING INSIGHT: This soup combines the anti-inflammatory properties of turmeric and ginger with the immune-supporting powers of garlic.

A study in the *Journal of Nutritional Biochemistry* found that curcumin (the active compound in turmeric) can modulate the immune system, potentially enhancing its ability to fight off pathogens.

APPENDIX B

NUTRIENT PROFILES OF 25 COMMON FOODS

This appendix provides a quick reference guide to the nutritional content of 25 common foods to help readers make informed choices about their diet and nutrient intake. For each food, I have included the serving size, calories, macronutrients, key vitamins and minerals, and special notes.

ALMONDS, RAW (1 OZ/28 G)
- ↷ Calories: 164
- ↷ Protein: 6g
- ↷ Fat: 14g (1.1g saturated)
- ↷ Carbohydrates: 6g (Fiber: 3.5g)
- ↷ Key nutrients:
    - o Vitamin E (7.3 mg)
    - o Magnesium (76 mg)
    - o Manganese (0.6 mg)
- ↷ Special notes: Good source of healthy fats and plant-based protein

AVOCADO (1/2 MEDIUM/100 G)
- ↷ Calories: 160
- ↷ Protein: 2g
- ↷ Fat: 14.7g (2.1g saturated)
- ↷ Carbohydrates: 8.5g (Fiber: 6.7g)
- ↷ Key nutrients:
    - o Vitamin K (21 mcg)
    - o Folate (81 mcg)
    - o Potassium (485 mg).
- ↷ Special notes: High in monounsaturated fats, potassium-rich.

BANANAS (1 MEDIUM/118 G)
- ↷ Calories: 105
- ↷ Protein: 1.3g
- ↷ Fat: 0.4g
- ↷ Carbohydrates: 27g (Fiber: 3.1g)
- ↷ Key nutrients:
    - o Vitamin C (10.3 mg)
    - o Potassium (422 mg)
    - o Vitamin B6 (0.4 mg)
- ↷ Special notes: Good source of resistant starch when unripe.

BEEF, GRASS-FED GROUND (3 OZ/85 G)

- Calories: 198
- Protein: 21g
- Fat: 12.7g (5.3g saturated)
- Carbohydrates: 0g
- Key nutrients:
    - Vitamin B12 (2.7 mcg)
    - Zinc (6 mg)
    - Iron (2.2 mg)
- Special notes: Higher in omega-3s compared to grain-fed beef.

BLUEBERRIES, RAW (1 CUP/148 G)

- Calories: 84
- Protein: 1.1g
- Fat: 0.5g
- Carbohydrates: 21g (Fiber: 3.6g)
- Key nutrients:
    - Vitamin C (14.4 mg)
    - Vitamin K (28.6 mg)
    - Manganese (0.5 mg)
- Special notes: High in antioxidants, especially anthocyanins.

BROCCOLI, RAW (1 CUP CHOPPED/91 G)

- Calories: 31
- Protein: 2.5g
- Fat: 0.3g
- Carbohydrates: 6g (Fiber: 2.4g)
- Key nutrients:
    - Vitamin C (81.2 mg)
    - Vitamin K (92.5 mcg)
    - Folate (57 mcg)
- Special notes: High in antioxidants and glucosinolates.

CHICKPEAS, COOKED (1 CUP/164 G)

- Calories: 269
- Protein: 14.5g
- Fat: 4.3g
- Carbohydrates: 45g (Fiber: 12.5g)
- Key nutrients:
  - Folate (282 mcg)
  - Manganese (1.7 mg)
  - Iron (4.7 mg)
- Special notes: Good source of plant-based protein and fiber.

DARK CHOCOLATE (70-85% COCOA) (1 OZ/28 G)

- Calories: 170
- Protein: 2.3g
- Fat: 12.1g (7.3g saturated)
- Carbohydrates: 13g (Fiber: 3.1g)
- Key nutrients:
  - Iron (3.4 mg)
  - Magnesium (64 mg)
  - Copper (0.5 mg)
- Special notes: High in antioxidants, especially flavonoids.

EGGS, LARGE, WHOLE (1 EGG / 50G)

- Calories: 72
- Protein: 6.3g
- Fat: 4.8g (1.6g saturated)
- Carbohydrates: 0.4g
- Key nutrients:
  - Vitamin A (270 IU)
  - Vitamin B12 (0.6 mcg)
  - Selenium (15.4 mcg)
- Special notes: Has all essential amino acids; source of choline.

GARLIC, RAW (1 CLOVE / 3 G)

- Calories: 4
- Protein: 0.2g
- Fat: 0g
- Carbohydrates: 1
- Key nutrients:
  - Vitamin C (0.9 mg)
  - Vitamin B6 (0.1 mg)
  - Manganese (0.2 mg)
- Special notes: Contains allicin, known for potential health benefits.

GINGER, GROUND (1 TEASPOON / 2 G)

- Calories: 6
- Protein: 0.2g
- Fat: 0.1g
- Carbohydrates: 1.3g
- Key nutrients:
  - Potassium (8.3 mg)
  - Magnesium (1.6 mg)
- Special notes: Contains gingerols, known for potential anti-inflammatory effects.

GREEK YOGURT, PLAIN, NON-FAT (6 OZ/170 G)

- Calories: 100
- Protein: 18g
- Fat: 0g
- Carbohydrates: 6g
- Key nutrients:
  - Calcium (200 mg)
  - Potassium (240 mg)
  - Vitamin B12 (1.3 mcg)
- Special notes: Probiotic food; high in protein.

GREEN TEA, BREWED (1 CUP (0.24 L) / 245 G)

- Calories: 2
- Protein: 0.5g
- Fat: 0g
- Carbohydrates: 0g
- Key nutrients:
  - o Lesser amounts of various minerals
- Special notes: Contains catechins, especially EGCG, known for potential health benefits.

KALE, RAW (1 CUP CHOPPED / 67G)

- Calories: 33
- Protein: 2.9g
- Fat: 0.6g
- Carbohydrates: 6.7g (Fiber: 1.3g)
- Key nutrients:
  - o Vitamin K (547 mcg)
  - o Vitamin C (80.4 mg)
  - o Vitamin A (10302 IU).
- Special notes: Very high in antioxidants and nutrients.

LENTILS, COOKED (1 CUP/198 G)

- Calories: 230
- Protein: 17.9g
- Fat: 0.8g
- Carbohydrates: 39.9g
- Fiber: 15.6g
- Key nutrients:
  - o Folate (358 mcg)
  - o Iron (6.6 mg)
  - o Magnesium (71 mg)
- Special notes: high in plant-based protein and fiber.

OATS, ROLLED (1/2 CUP DRY/40 G)

- Calories: 150
- Protein: 5g
- Fat: 3g
- Carbohydrates: 27g
- Fiber: 4g
- Key nutrients:
  - Manganese (1.9 mg)
  - Phosphorus (180 mg)
  - Thiamine (0.2 mg)
- Special notes: Contains beta-glucan, beneficial for heart health.

OLIVE OIL (1 TABLESPOON / 13.5 G)

- Calories: 119
- Protein: 0g
- Fat: 13.5g
- Saturated Fat: 1.9g
- Carbohydrates: 0g
- Key nutrients:
  - Vitamin E (1.9 mg)
  - Vitamin K (8.1 mcg)
- Special notes: High in monounsaturated fats, holds polyphenols.

QUINOA, COOKED (1 CUP/185 G)

- Calories: 222
- Protein: 8g
- Fat: 3.6g
- Carbohydrates: 39g
- Fiber: 5.2g
- Key nutrients:
  - Magnesium (118 mg)
  - Phosphorus (281 mg)
  - Folate (77.7 mcg)

- ✿ Special notes: Complete protein source, gluten-free.

SALMON (ATLANTIC, FARMED), COOKED (3 OZ/85 G)

- ✿ Calories: 175
- ✿ Protein: 19g
- ✿ Fat: 11g
- ✿ Saturated Fat: 1.9g
- ✿ Carbohydrates: 0g
- ✿ Key nutrients:
  - o Vitamin D (447 IU)
  - o Vitamin B12 (2.6 mcg)
  - o Selenium (26 mcg)
- ✿ Special notes: Excellent source of omega-3 fatty acids.

SPINACH, RAW (1 CUP/30 G)

- ✿ Calories: 7
- ✿ Protein: 0.9g
- ✿ Fat: 0.1g
- ✿ Carbohydrates: 1.1g
- ✿ Fiber: 0.7g
- ✿ Key nutrients:
  - o Vitamin K (145 mcg)
  - o Vitamin A (2813 IU)
  - o Folate (58.2 mcg)
- ✿ Special notes: High in antioxidants, especially lutein and zeaxanthin.

SWEET POTATO, BAKED WITH SKIN (1 MEDIUM/114 G)

- ✿ Calories: 103
- ✿ Protein: 2.3g
- ✿ Fat: 0.2g
- ✿ Carbohydrates: 23.6g
- ✿ Fiber: 3.8g
- ✿ Key nutrients:
  - o Vitamin A (21907 IU)

- o Vitamin C (22.3 mg)
- o Manganese (0.6 mg)
- ⚕ Special notes: High in beta-carotene, a precursor to Vitamin A.

TURMERIC, GROUND (1 TEASPOON / 2.8 G)
- ⚕ Calories: 9
- ⚕ Protein: 0.3g
- ⚕ Fat: 0.1g
- ⚕ Carbohydrates: 2g
- ⚕ Key nutrients:
  - o Iron (1.6 mg)
  - o Manganese (0.2 mg)
- ⚕ Special notes: Contains curcumin, known for anti-inflammatory properties.

WALNUTS (1 OZ/28 G)
- ⚕ Calories: 185
- ⚕ Protein: 4.3g
- ⚕ Fat: 18.5g
- ⚕ Saturated fat: 1.7g
- ⚕ Carbohydrates: 3.9g
- ⚕ Fiber: 1.9g
- ⚕ Key nutrients:
  - o Manganese (0.9 mg)
  - o Copper (0.4 mg)
- ⚕ Special notes: High in omega-3 fatty acids (plant-based ALA).

BIBLIOGRAPHY

Chandalia, M, et al. "Beneficial Effects of High Dietary Fiber Intake in Patients with Type 2 Diabetes Mellitus." *The New England Journal of Medicine*, U.S. National Library of Medicine, 11 May 2000, pubmed.ncbi.nlm.nih.gov/10805824/.

Chang, Yuwen, et al. "Time-Restricted Eating Improves Health Because of Energy Deficit and Circadian Rhythm: A Systematic Review and Meta-Analysis." *iScience*, U.S. National Library of Medicine, 26 Jan. 2024, pmc.ncbi.nlm.nih.gov/articles/PMC10865403/.

Del Bo', Cristian, et al. "Systematic Review on Polyphenol Intake and Health Outcomes: Is There Sufficient Evidence to Define a Health-Promoting Polyphenol-Rich Dietary Pattern?" *MDPI*, Multidisciplinary Digital Publishing Institute, 16 June 2019, www.mdpi.com/2072-6643/11/6/1355.

Estruch, Ramón, et al. "Primary Prevention of Cardiovascular Disease with a Mediterranean Diet Supplemented with Extra-Virgin Olive Oil or Nuts." *The New England Journal of Medicine*, U.S. National Library of Medicine, 21 June 2018, pubmed.ncbi.nlm.nih.gov/29897866/.

Kim, Hyunju, et al. "Plant-based Diets Are Associated with a Lower Risk of Incident Cardiovascular Disease, Cardiovascular Disease Mortality, and All-cause Mortality in a General Population of Middle-aged Adults | Journal of the American Heart Association." *JAHA - Journal of the American Heart Association*, American Heart Association, 7 Aug. 2019, www.ahajournals.org/doi/10.1161/JAHA.119.012865.

Lane, Melissa M, et al. "Ultra-Processed Food Exposure and Adverse Health Outcomes: Umbrella Review of Epidemiological Meta-Analyses." *BMJ (Clinical Research Ed.)*, U.S. National Library of Medicine, 24 Feb. 2024, pubmed.ncbi.nlm.nih.gov/38418082/.

Liu, Di, et al. "Vitamin D and Multiple Health Outcomes: An Umbrella Review of Observational Studies, Randomized Controlled Trials, and Mendelian Randomization Studies." *Advances in Nutrition (Bethesda, Md.)*, U.S. National Library of Medicine, 1 Aug. 2022, pubmed.ncbi.nlm.nih.gov/34999745/.

Martineau, Adrian R, et al. "Vitamin D Supplementation to Prevent Acute Respiratory Tract Infections: Systematic Review and Meta-Analysis of Individual Participant Data." *BMJ (Clinical Research Ed.)*, U.S. National Library of Medicine, 15 Feb. 2017, pubmed.ncbi.nlm.nih.gov/28202713/.

Morris, Martha Clare, et al. "Mind Diet Associated with Reduced Incidence of Alzheimer's Disease." *Alzheimer's & Dementia : The Journal of the Alzheimer's Association*, U.S. National Library of Medicine, 11 Sept. 2015, pubmed.ncbi.nlm.nih.gov/25681666/.

Njike, Valentine Yanchou, et al. "Snack Food, Satiety, and Weight." *Advances in Nutrition (Bethesda, Md.)*, U.S. National Library of Medicine, 15 Sept. 2015, www.ncbi.nlm.nih.gov/pmc/articles/PMC5015032/.

Pagliai, G, et al. "Consumption of Ultra-Processed Foods and Health Status: A Systematic Review and Meta-Analysis." *The British Journal of Nutrition*, U.S. National Library of Medicine, 14 Feb. 2021, pubmed.ncbi.nlm.nih.gov/32792031/.

Panda, Satchidananda, et al. "Time-Restricted Eating for the Prevention and Management of Metabolic Diseases | Endocrine Reviews | Oxford Academic." *Endocrine Reviews*, Oxford University Press, 1 Apr. 2022, academic.oup.com/edrv/article/43/2/405/6371193.

Rasenberg, Marloo, et al. "The Multimodal Nature of Communicative Efficiency in Social Interaction." *Scientific Reports*, U.S. National Library of Medicine, 9 Nov. 2022, pubmed.ncbi.nlm.nih.gov/36351949/.

Rebholz, Casey M, et al. "Plant-based Diets Are Associated with a Lower Risk of Incident Cardiovascular Disease, Cardiovascular Disease Mortality, and All-cause Mortality in a General Population of Middle-aged Adults | Journal of the American Heart Association." *JAHA - Journal of the American Heart Association*, American Heart Association, 7 Aug. 2019, www.ahajournals.org/doi/10.1161/JAHA.119.012865.

Reynolds, Andrew N, et al. "Dietary Fibre and Whole Grains in Diabetes Management: Systematic Review and Meta-Analyses." *PLoS Medicine*, U.S. National Library of Medicine, 6 Mar. 2020, pubmed.ncbi.nlm.nih.gov/32142510/.

Singh, Rasnik K, et al. "Influence of Diet on the Gut Microbiome and Implications for Human Health." *Journal of Translational Medicine*, U.S. National

Library of Medicine, 8 Apr. 2017, pub-med.ncbi.nlm.nih.gov/28388917/.

Sutton, Elizabeth F, et al. "Early Time-Restricted Feeding Improves Insulin Sensitivity, Blood Pressure, and Oxidative Stress Even without Weight Loss in Men with Prediabetes." *Cell Metabolism*, U.S. National Library of Medicine, 5 June 2018, pubmed.ncbi.nlm.nih.gov/29754952/.

Veronese, Nicola, et al. "Magnesium and Health Outcomes: An Umbrella Review of Systematic Reviews and Meta-Analyses of Observational and Intervention Studies." *European Journal of Nutrition*, U.S. National Library of Medicine, 1 Feb. 2020, pubmed.ncbi.nlm.nih.gov/30684032/.

Wang, Yeli, et al. "Associations between Plant-Based Dietary Patterns and Risks of Type 2 Diabetes, Cardiovascular Disease, Cancer, and Mortality - A Systematic Review and Meta-Analysis." *Nutrition Journal*, U.S. National Library of Medicine, 4 Oct. 2023, pub-med.ncbi.nlm.nih.gov/37789346/.

Witte, A Veronica, et al. "Long-Chain Omega-3 Fatty Acids Improve Brain Function and Structure in Older Adults." *Cerebral Cortex (New York, N.Y. : 1991)*, U.S. National Library of Medicine, 24 Nov. 2014, pub-med.ncbi.nlm.nih.gov/23796946/.

Yancy, William S, et al. "A Low-Carbohydrate, Ketogenic Diet to Treat Type 2 Diabetes." *Nutrition & Metabolism*, U.S. National Library of Medicine, 1 Dec. 2005, pubmed.ncbi.nlm.nih.gov/16318637/.

www.ingramcontent.com/pod-product-compliance
Lightning Source LLC
Chambersburg PA
CBHW061739120626
46550CB00005B/1828